Birth International

"Humanising birth through the protection, promotion and support of midwifery"

Publishers of these best-selling titles
by Andrea Robertson

"Empowering Women"
- Teaching Active Birth

"The Midwife Companion"
- The art of support during birth

"Preparing For Birth: Mothers"

"Preparing For Birth: Fathers"

*View our complete range of books, videos,
charts, models, teaching aids and accessories:*

www.birthinternational.com

Secure online ordering

Birth International
PO Box 366, Camperdown NSW Australia 1450

EMPOWERING WOMEN

Teaching Active Birth

Andrea Robertson

Published by Birth International
PO Box 366
Camperdown NSW 1450
Australia
Phone: +61 2 9564 2322
Fax: +61 2 9564 2388
email: sales@birthinternational.com
www.birthinternational.com

First Published 1994
Reprinted 1997,1999
Reprinted 2002
Reprinted 2003

ISBN 0 646 16836 3

Printed in Australia by McPherson's Printing Group
Cover design by S2 Design
Text design and layout by Step Two Designs

PREFACE

The pace of change within childbirth education has quickened in the past five years. Once we concentrated on teaching our clients how to breathe and relax during labour, and gave advice on baby care and breastfeeding. Now we are beginning to recognise that childbirth education is grounded in a process, not in specific content, and we are starting to apply to this area of adult education the principles and practices used in other areas of effective adult learning.

The application of scientific rigour to the evaluation of medical technologies and practices used in birth has put considerable pressure on everyone involved in maternity care. Childbirth educators must be familiar with the latest research, in addition to retaining their understanding of the normal birth process. The physiology of labour and birth receive little attention as the spotlight is turned on the multitude of obstetric procedures that need to be assessed, yet having a firm grasp of normal physiology, and the ability to explain it to others, forms the foundation for empowering women.

When I set out to revise *Teaching Active Birth* in readiness for the production of a new edition, I realised that there was so much I now wanted to add that a new book was required. Since writing the original text in 1987-88, I myself had undergone much personal development in the field of childbirth education, and I wanted to share this experience with my colleagues.

Whilst I have been involved in the training of childbirth educators since developing the first training course in Australia in 1977, the last five years have given me new perspectives, stemming primarily from my commitment to have the training course properly accredited. The National Training Board, established by the Australian Government, offered this opportunity. This innovative scheme enables providers of independent educational courses to have their programs evaluated and recognised in the same way as those offered through existing tertiary training institutions. The work involved, and in particular the need to be very specific in describing the role and scope of childbirth education, both for the students doing the course and for their clients, has proved an invaluable learning experience. Having the course accredited as a Graduate Diploma in Childbirth Education is exciting and, I feel, finally puts this emerging profession on the map within the health care system in Australia.

With each revision of the training course I have valued the input and generosity of other childbirth educators, who have stimulated new thoughts and forced me to remain flexible. During the last review, which ultimately led to the accreditation of the course, I have been particularly indebted to Hilary

Tupling, who as my co-tutor for many training workshops, always challenged me to evaluate my work as a trainer and whose style of teaching left many messages about adult learning embedded in my unconscious brain. At times it was hard, but it has always been invaluable.

Books such as these never get written without much practical help and assistance. In particular Lee Marshall made sure it was all English, and James Robertson ensured it would be attractive and readable in its final printed form. As usual my staff have provided much support and encouragement from the sidelines.

My aim in writing this book is to assist all educators to revise and review the work they are doing, whether they have been teaching for some time or are just beginning to develop their program. On many occasions, educators just need some new ideas or fresh insights to help them revamp their classes. New educators need to be able to draw on the experience of others as they begin to plan their own presentations. I hope that this book will fulfil both of these needs in a practical, straightforward manner.

Andrea Robertson
February 1994

CONTENTS

PART TWO
EXPLORING ANATOMY AND PHYSIOLOGY

PART THREE
TEACHING ACTIVITIES FOR CLASSES

PART 4
PUTTING IT ALL TOGETHER

CHAPTER 9
DESIGNING YOUR PRE-NATAL CLASSES

Introduction

The formal organisation and presentation of childbirth education classes is a western concept that has been with us now for over 50 years. Traditionally, pregnant women learned about birth and the nurturing of babies from observation of their extended families, tribal or cultural lore and information passed on by close female relatives, and the ministrations of the midwife who provided support and specific care during the pregnancy, birth and post partum period.

The removal of birth from the seclusion and protection of the home and family and its placement in the mysterious, clinical and unfamiliar territory of the hospital has completely disrupted the natural educational process of this traditional social setting. As birth became steeped in a medical flavour, its management based on the notion that technology and external guidance in a hospital would give better results, traditional childbirth education became inadequate. Pregnant women found themselves facing birth with little idea of what would happen and few social supports within a health care system that focused more on its own needs rather than on the needs of the woman herself or her family.

Grantly Dick-Read was one of the first physicians to notice the effect of this medicalisation on the birth process itself: women were labouring longer and having more painful and difficult births. He concluded that education may provide a key to improving women's experiences, reasoning that if they were better informed and therefore less frightened the normal physiological responses to fear would be reduced and birth would proceed more smoothly. His solution was, however, based on the medical model. Instead of recognising the need for more appropriate social settings for birth, he suggested organised classes where women were taught how to respond to contractions. Instead of trusting their instincts and reviving physiological methods to ease the pain, women were subjected to patronising instructions that, although offered with the best of intentions and a genuine desire to help, missed the basic point: women are born with the innate ability to give birth, and the best course of action is to strenuously avoid any disturbance of this normal bodily function.

From these humble beginnings, a childbirth education industry evolved, especially in western countries, paralleling the technical, medical takeover of birth by doctors and the demise of midwives and home birth. At the same time, the disruptions to family life caused by war, changes in employment patterns, migration, the evolution of new family structures and the assertion of women's rights all contributed to a lack of social support for pregnant women and reduced educational opportunities within the extended family and community. Pregnant western women today are confronted by a bewildering array of medical technology, are pressured to give birth in a hospital, lack family and community support and live in a culture in which birth is viewed as a risky and difficult process.

In this climate, childbirth education has become an essential part of pre-natal care for the majority of first time mothers and their partners. With few opportunities for learning from each other, or from experienced relatives or a personal midwife, women have instead chosen to attend formal classes to learn about birth and parenting. Many hospitals and community groups have risen to the challenge of providing education classes, with mixed success.

Initially, the emphasis in these classes was on training women for birth, and in providing advice on child rearing. Several methods were devised as a basis for the training — psychoprophylaxis, 'Lamaze' and the 'Bradley Method' became well known. Structured breathing and relaxation form the basis of these methods (without any scientific evidence that they are effective or even safe) and a successful birth (read 'pain free') was promised if the method was followed rigorously. Although based on a genuine desire to help women survive, both physically and emotionally, a potentially traumatic labour and birth in the most inappropriate of settings, the medical model that labels women as patients in need of diagnosis and treatment forms the basis of this approach. Birth classes could thus be described as a form of intervention in their own right.

The gradual rise of consumerism within the community over the past 20 years has affected health care. A new theme began to emerge in childbirth education: the need for parents to make informed choice about birth options and the necessity for a wider range of information to be made available to prospective parents so that appropriate decisions could be properly made. Until the early 80's, this approach did not extend to the actual methods being taught in classes, and psychoprophylaxis (and its derivatives) continued unchallenged. Indeed, in some countries, the new consumerism took an interesting twist, with an expansion of the breathing and relaxation methods being introduced on the basis that this allowed parents to make a 'choice' between methods! The option of abandoning proscribed behaviours in favour of encouraging natural and personal responses to labour, has still not been considered in some western countries. The business of childbirth education can have vested interests too.

In the early 80's a new philosophy for childbirth education emerged, based largely on observations of women giving birth in the familiar and protective atmosphere of their own homes. It was noticed that these women used a variety of means to manage their labour and that pain killing drugs were rarely used. The innate behaviours, born of instinct and hormonal physiology, seemed sufficient in themselves for pain management during birth, and the results were often spectacular and exciting, especially for care givers used to witnessing the aftermath of birth in hospital settings. These mothers and babies were contented and physically well, and the women were elated and exalted by their achievement. Altogether, this was an ideal emotional climate in which to begin the nurturing of the new baby.

This new approach to childbirth preparation was termed 'active birth'. The expression was originally coined by Janet Balaskas, who used it to counter the medical 'active management of labour' that was prevalent at the time. As the concept grew and was adapted to local conditions, it came to be defined not as a birth preparation method, but more as a philosophic approach to birth. Briefly, the essence of active birth could be summarised as a birth in which:

- a woman labours instinctively, following her own physiological rhythms and responses,
- the woman takes responsibility for arranging an appropriate setting and caregivers who will enable her to labour as she needs when the time comes,
- the woman, and her partner, are involved in all aspects of pregnancy and birth care, and are enabled to make informed decisions whenever necessary,
- management of the labour is rooted in the midwifery rather than the medical model,
- it is assumed by all involved that the labour and birth are normal, until there is conclusive medical evidence of a problem,
- the woman's assessment of the outcome is accepted and used as the primary measure of success or satisfaction, rather than evaluations made by her caregivers.

An active birth could also be described as one in which the woman is empowered to give birth using her own resources and abilities. In simple terms, a person is empowered when they take control over what happens to them. In practice, for a woman to feel empowered within our maternity care system suggests that a number of principles are in place:

- she is fully aware of her rights and responsibilities,
- she is enabled to exercise her rights and make decisions about care affecting herself and her baby,
- she has the necessary social supports to ensure her physical and emotional well being,

- she is not subject to discrimination based on her age, sex or her state of pregnancy,
- her ability to grow, produce and nurture her baby is respected and accepted within the framework of birth as a normal bodily function for women.

These philosophies have led to the development of a different kind of pre-natal class, where the emphasis is on enabling the parents to develop appropriate skills necessary for obtaining the kind of birth they desire and need. Instead of giving advice and information in didactic teaching sessions, a more flexible approach based on the individual parent's goals, practical problem solving and the development of communication and negotiating abilities has evolved. Rather than seeing the birth itself as an end point for education, it is viewed as one step in the process of becoming a parent, and an opportunity for practising skills that will be useful after the baby is born.

There are many obstacles for a woman to overcome before she can feel empowered during her pregnancy. The entrenched medical model of care firmly places the onus of responsibility on the caregiver rather than on the parents. The fear of litigation has ensured that risk assessments, management plans, protocols, procedures and practical care have all developed with the caregiver's needs as the foremost consideration, even though they are ostensibly in place to protect the mother and baby.

The plethora of technological interventions with their inherent jargon is difficult to understand, and at times there seems to be conspiracy to withhold vital information from women, especially about the scientific validity of many tests and procedures. This smacks of discrimination and can be a deliberate ploy by the physician to retain power.

The need to develop systems for the delivery of health care to a whole population has meant that individual needs are sacrificed in the name of expediency. Women are classified, treated and managed according to a set of averages instead of being recognised and accepted as individuals with special needs unique to each mother and baby pair.

Care givers and policy makers have been slow to accept the social nature of birth. The needs of pregnant women, particularly for emotional support and decent living conditions have largely been overlooked. It may be impossible for women to feel empowered when they are dealing with inadequate housing, a lack of finance or an absence of family supports.

Given these hurdles to empowerment for women during pregnancy (and there are no doubt many more that could have been included in the list), what role can childbirth education play in enabling women and their partners to get a better deal?

In an ideal world, every pregnant woman would be assisted and supported through her pregnancy and birth by her own personal midwife. There would be little need for formal gatherings to learn specifically about birth and parenting, since a woman's needs and questions would be addressed by the midwife on an individual basis. There would still be a place for informal gatherings of pregnant women, to make social contact, share experiences and provide mutual support. Since our health care system does not generally provide for continuity of care by a personal midwife, women have turned increasingly to a new health professional — the childbirth educator, for information and the opportunity for social contact with other expectant parents.

The growth of childbirth education, to fill this void in our health care system, has been phenomenal, and today most maternity hospitals provide pre-natal classes and many community based groups also offer parenthood education programs. As a result, instead of the midwife being the most consistently available health professional for a pregnant woman, it is the childbirth educator who spends most hours with individual mothers during the pregnancy. In some centres this even extends to the labour itself, and it is the childbirth educator who continues the support during the birth.

Until extensive midwifery programs are in place, the childbirth educator therefore has a very important role to play in the lives of pregnant women. It is the educator who will spend the most time with the pregnant woman and her partner, who will be the primary source of information about maternity services and birth options, who can initiate social contacts between pregnant women within the community and who can assist parents to become empowered within the system. It is an important and challenging role.

In this context, pre-natal classes based in the community and presented independently of hospital settings have always had one major advantage — they are not subject to those political pressures that exist within a hospital system. Therefore, the educators have been able to design their presentation to reflect a consumer perspective with less fear of reprisal from employers.

The true worth of good quality pre-natal education is only beginning to be recognised, both within and outside childbirth education circles. Since Grantly Dick-Read first co-opted physiotherapists to run some pre-natal groups in addition to their normal caseload, the work of the childbirth educator has been regarded by hospital based personnel as an 'extra' within the job description of a health professional, usually a midwife. Hospital administrators have often had the attitude that if a person is qualified as a midwife or physiotherapist then running the classes should easily fall within their expertise. It is ironic that new parents often complain that raising children is the one job for which they receive no training, yet the same could be said of pre-natal educators since adult education methods, teaching skills and group leadership are not usually part of the training of the health professionals charged with conducting the classes. Most have tried valiantly to provide effective education, perhaps because they have instinctively empathised with the needs of the people in their groups. Some have become very skilled, largely through self-education and intuition rather than through specific training programs. The chances of a skilled educator being available however, are rather small, and it is no wonder that many of the research projects designed to evaluate the effectiveness of childbirth education have offered very mixed results. With no consistent approach to classes, no formal training of the pre-natal group leaders, no consensus on what constitutes useful content, it is not surprising that the outcomes of childbirth education are equivocal.

What makes a good childbirth educator?

Effective childbirth educators are those who have developed the same qualities and skills as effective parents and who, in addition, have a theoretical and practical grounding developed through training and experience appropriate for their profession. They are able to model the behaviours parents themselves need: self-awareness, resourcefulness, flexibility, problem-solving abilities, stress management, good communication, negotiating skills and sensitivity. Many of these qualities have developed from their own experiences as parents, although this is not necessarily a pre-requisite for an adult educator. Good training, however, is necessary, as it is for any member of the health care team. Some educators develop their skills through on-the-job training, having been thrust into the position of presenting classes with little or no preparation. Just as some parents can manage to learn parent craft through trial and error with their own children, and many find it a struggle (sometimes with unfortunate results for their children), some childbirth educators are able to gradually learn, from their clients, what it takes to present useful pre-natal classes. This is haphazard, at best, and unprofessional, at worst.

There is no substitute for good, basic training in the theory of adult education and the practical development of skills under the supervision of a mentor and guide. This book is intended to provide some of the background theory and a framework on which practical skills can be developed.

As you read through the early chapters, the broad picture of working with adults will unfold. The micro skills that you need to develop yourself will come with further reading and practical experience. These can best be obtained in workshop settings where you can practise amongst colleagues before embarking on parent groups.

The anatomy and physiology of labour is a fascinating subject, centred as it is on the creative and adaptive responses of individual women in labour. Again, these chapters are designed to tickle your curiosity and inspire you to learn more from being with women during the greatest adventure of their lives. Developing a healthy, holistic, trusting attitude towards the immense power and capabilities of women takes experience and sensitivity. By pulling some of the major themes in this story together, I have aimed to lay the groundwork for your explorations in this area.

Teaching is more than just taking an activity off a 'shelf' and presenting it to a group, as I hope you will discover from reading Part 3. There are many more possible activities for pre-natal classes that could have been included, and this selection revolves around the basic theme of enabling women to feel empowered through birth.

Part 4 describes some of the processes involved in establishing your classes and setting up a system for ongoing evaluation that will enable you to develop as an educator. Planning takes time and thought and leads to feelings of confidence and being organised, which are helpful in any life setting.

Working to empower others is extraordinarily rewarding. Working to empower pregnant women as they strive to fulfil their potential through birth is a privilege and pleasure, with profound yet subtle benefits for you as a person. I trust that the theoretical background in this book will inspire your own journey of discovery through the opportunity to share a corner of the lives of the expectant and new parents with whom you will be working. Practice and experience will add to your education. Best wishes for your travels!

PART ONE

BEFORE YOU BEGIN

Chapter 1

Your teaching plan

When you are developing your teaching plan for pre-natal classes, it helps to take a broad view of your purpose. Pre-natal classes are sometimes called 'Preparation for Parenthood' classes, which is in many ways more accurate. In the past, the emphasis in classes was to impart information and give advice. Explaining hospital policy and procedures was also high on the list of objectives for educators. If we take the broader view, however, what we are really doing is working with people making the transition to parenthood, and this is a process that is easier for parents if they have specific skills, such as:

- an ability to solve problems and make decisions,
- knowledge of resources and how they can be used,
- stress management techniques,
- flexibility in their approach and thinking,
- confidence in their competence as parents,
- an ability to recognise their limitations.

If new parents possessed these skills and abilities, then caring for their new baby, especially the first child, would be much less stressful and much more enjoyable. Most adults will have some or all of these skills which they use in other areas of their lives. One of our roles as educators can be to help them apply these abilities to parenting. Since people become parents as soon as a baby is conceived, it makes sense to start using them to work out the myriad problems and situations that will occur during the pregnancy and labour. These can be regarded as 'full dress rehearsals' which provide many valuable opportunities for practice.

Keep these skills in mind when you are developing your aims and objectives. The activities, exercises and discussions you plan for your class should all fit this broader agenda of empowering parents through enabling them to develop these parenting skills.

It takes time and effort to develop a comprehensive teaching plan, and many educators avoid doing this advance planning. Instead, they use a plan developed by another educator, or the guidelines issued by their employer, or just base their classes on what they learned themselves from classes and their own births. As a trainer of childbirth educators, I receive many requests for the 'formula' for classes, preferably set out week by week, so that the inquirer can take the format and begin teaching without needing to do any preparation. These educators may feel annoyed by my apparent lack of co-operation, but I know that using someone else's teaching plan is risky for an educator, apart from being unprofessional.

There are many benefits to be gained from taking the time to thoroughly plan your classes and develop a set of clear educational objectives for your teaching. Such a plan:

- sets out a clear overview of the purpose of the class series and provides overall direction,
- describes exactly what you are doing and why,
- simplifies on-going planning, as you have a framework in place, which can easily be altered,
- increases your flexibility as an educator as you will have a list of various ways to present any topic, and can choose accordingly,
- assists in the marketing of your classes as it describes what clients can expect to learn from attending your group,
- provides you with a model that can assist clients formulate their own aims and objectives,
- provides inbuilt methods for evaluation and assessment of the effectiveness of your teaching,
- boosts your confidence, through being well organised,
- describes the ways in which you can empower your clients, and provides a reminder that their needs are paramount.

Having a set of aims and objectives will also help you avoid some of the common traps for childbirth educators:

- not knowing what you are going to teach or why you are doing it,
- feeling 'out of control' when the group deviates from the topic,
- being surprised when the group reacts in an unexpected way to your presentation,
- being unable to identify exactly what your clients have learned in your class,
- teaching the same way all the time to try and make it easier — 'if this is Wednesday, then it must be a Week 3'.
- knowing that your message is not getting through, but not knowing how to improve it,
- feeling bored and burnt out through lack of stimulation and appreciation,

- feeling hurt when group members offer negative feedback on their evaluations,
- using your client's birth experience as a measure of the success of your teaching.

Therefore, instead of, for example, measuring success by how many couples use pain killing drugs in labour, try rating your classes by measuring satisfaction with the class series, the social networks formed in the group, or the demonstrated ability of our group members to describe the choices available to them in a given situation. If parents can show they know how to make a decision or solve a problem, this is an excellent educational outcome for group sessions. The actual decisions they make in labour will depend on the circumstances at the time and will reflect their assessment of that situation. The important thing is that they have the skills to make the decision in the first

TABLE 1: *Initial planning: sorting out your objectives and those of your clients.*

Some educator objectives	Possible client objectives
Explain choices and options	Obtain information
Provide social contacts and facilitate networking	Meet other parents
Give unbiased scientific information	Learn about baby care
Act as a resource person	Labour ward tour
Be available for individuals when needed	See a video of birth
Be a support person	Learn coping skills for labour
Meet client's needs	Find out about breastfeeding
Present information appropriately for client's learning styles	Have specific questions answered
Communicate effectively	Learn about choices and options
Evaluate outcome of the classes	Find out what happens in hospital
Appropriate use of teaching aids	Learn how to be a "good" parent

place, and that these are skills that can be reinforced or developed in pre-natal groups.

The two agendas

When you begin this planning process, you need to be aware that there are two sets of aims and objectives to be considered — yours as the group leader or educator, and those of your clients or group participants. Of these, the needs of your clients or the group (their goals and objectives) are the most important. Assisting your clients to achieve their desired outcomes for the birth or parenting, is, after all, the primary purpose of your work. Therefore the main focus of your planning must be on finding ways to meet their needs.

Of course, you have your own set of aims and objectives too, some directed at your own needs as an educator, some geared towards the practicalities of presenting classes or leading groups and others describing strategies for meeting your client's goals.

As an educator, you have a responsibility to meet not only your own aims and objectives, but also those of your client or group, including enabling them to meet some of their own goals. It is a very full agenda, and may seem overwhelming at first glance, but with planning it all becomes much clearer and achievable.

What are aims, objectives and outcomes?

Aims

Aims are global in nature. They are a statement of what is to be achieved overall, either by the end of the series or at the end of each class or topic. An aim is a statement of purpose that gives broad direction and scope. Examples of aims for pre-natal classes:

- 'To provide opportunities for group members to mix socially and develop support networks' (an aim for the educator).
- 'To provide a supportive environment in which group members can discuss issues of importance to them' (an aim for the educator, based on clients' needs).
- 'To provide information that will assist parents make informed decisions about maternity care' (an aim based on clients' needs).

- 'To arrange a series of practical sessions to explore self help ideas for increasing comfort in labour' (an aim for the educator).

Aims do not spell out how they will be achieved, therefore each aim will need a number of objectives that describe the series of actions that will be taken in order to achieve the aim.

OBJECTIVES

An objective describes what the client or the educator will be doing to help achieve the aim. Objectives describe behaviours which can be measured and they are therefore able to be evaluated because the results can be observed.

Objectives may relate to either the client's needs or those of the educator. It is relatively easy to identify your own objectives as these will be linked to the overall purpose of the classes and the educational outcomes desired for your clients. Group members, however, do not always have a clear idea of what they expect to achieve from classes, beyond simple statements such as 'to learn about birth'. As you stimulate discovery and curiosity about birth and parenting, group members may realise that there are other things they want to know or skills they wish to develop, and, as a result, they will be able to develop further objectives of their own.

An example: A mother may state that she is coming to class to learn about pain relief for labour. This is her *aim* — to find out what she can do to ease her pain in labour. Her *objective* may be to learn about self help measures and available drugs to make her labour more comfortable. When, as part of a group activity, she demonstrates various positions for labour, describes her 'goody bag' of comfort aids and names three available pain-killing drugs, you know that she has achieved her objective, and therefore her aim.

For your part, you will have another set of aims and objectives for her. Your aim will be to meet her need for information, and to provide her with a range of choices and options she can consider for pain relief. Specific objectives, however, might include:

- 'to provide a list of potential pain relief measures for use in labour',
- 'to explain the advantages and disadvantages of each measure' and
- 'to provide opportunities to practise problem solving exercises involving management of pain in labour'.

Your client didn't specifically ask for help with problem solving, but as an educator you know that just having the information is not usually enough to empower parents, and that they need to practise making decisions to function effectively during labour. Similarly, your client didn't ask you to list the advantages and disadvantages of each option, but you know that they need this information if they are to make an informed choice.

The objectives set out in the above example, such as 'to provide a list', describe behaviours, which can be observed as part of the evaluation process. In this case, if you have given the group a list, you have achieved your objective.

You will notice that there are no objectives, in this example, that relate to the outcome of the actual birth. Even though you may fervently hope that your client can manage the pain of labour using non-invasive self-help measures, it is unrealistic to have an objective that states, for example 'to reduce the rate of epidural use through better preparation for birth'. If this objective is to be achieved, your client will have to forgo an epidural in labour, which places the onus on her to fulfil your objective for you. In other words, if she selects an epidural, you have failed to achieve your objective. This is not only poor educational practice (you must take responsibility for fulfilling your own objectives) it is also unconscionable to place clients in a position of 'passing or failing' depending on their behaviour as measured against your objectives. This kind of objective also implies that you have a belief (that epidural use is too high/should be reduced/is 'bad') that is more important than the views and needs of your client during labour.

WRITING OBJECTIVES

When preparing your written objectives keep in mind that they must:

- Describe behaviours that are measurable. Another way of expressing this, is to ask yourself 'what will my client/group be doing, when they are fulfilling this objective? What will I see or hear when they are completing this task?'
- Begin with a suitable verb, for example: list, describe, participate, practise, draw, demonstrate, and so on. (Be wary of 'understand', 'increase awareness', 'couples will know'. These are impossible to measure — how do people behave when they understand? How do you assess awareness?)
- Be written in the positive, to foster empowering behaviours.
- Be realistic and achievable. 'Renegotiate hospital policy regarding electronic fetal monitoring' may be a worthy objective, but it unrealistic for parents to undertake!

Here are some examples:

AIM

✓ 'To provide opportunities for group members to mix socially and to develop support networks' (This is an aim for the educator's agenda).

OBJECTIVES FOR THIS AIM

* Provide a refreshment break of 20 minutes during the class.
* Compile a list, with the permission of the group, of the names, addresses and phone numbers of the group members, to be distributed within the group.
* Begin each of the first three classes with an introduction game or ice-breaker activity to assist group members to learn each other's names.

AIM

✓ 'To provide information that will assist parents wishing to make informed decisions about options in maternity care' (an aim based on clients' expressed needs).

OBJECTIVES FOR THIS AIM

(There are many possible objectives for this broad aim — here are some that tackle it from one viewpoint).

* Provide a copy of *Preparing for Birth* to each mother in the group.
* Having allowed time for the relevant section in *Preparing for Birth* on Obstetric Drugs and Interventions to be studied, group members will arrange a list of advantages and disadvantages of epidurals, pethidine and nitrous oxide and oxygen under the appropriate headings.
* Having participated in a discussion on the process of making decisions, group members will practise this skill using a number of cards describing labour situations where the use of pain killing drugs could be considered.

In each of the above examples it will be easy to evaluate if the objective has been met. You will be able to tell if you have 'provided a refreshment break' or 'made a list and distributed it' or 'provided a copy of *Preparing for Birth*. You can also tell if group members have correctly identified the advantages and disadvantages of epidurals or 'practised making decisions'. Thus it will be easy to assess the effectiveness of your work and the educational value of your program. It will also help you identify times when your message was not clear, or where learning was not complete. This can help you improve your teaching.

Objectives may relate to the class series as a whole, a particular session in the series or a topic. For example:

- 'To provide information about pain relief in labour'. This is an objective relating to the series as a whole.
- 'To describe and demonstrate self-help measures for pain relief in the first stage of labour'. This is an objective for a specific class in the series.
- 'To list the advantages and disadvantages of epidurals'. This objective describes a specific topic within the class.

All of these may be grouped under the overall aim of 'discussion on choices and options in labour and birth'.

Some objectives will be related to specific teaching strategies. For example:

- 'Using a set of cards that describe the advantages and disadvantages of epidurals, arrange them in two groups — those that relate to the baby and those that affect the mother.' This is an objective for a particular teaching activity, and describes the way in which the topic objective will be achieved.

When you are preparing your aims and objectives, it is helpful to write your aims as an overview and to prepare a series of objectives that are both specific for each aim and wide in their application. Devising a number of objectives that describe a variety of teaching activities will help you define your presentation strategies and give you a range of activities from which you can make appropriate selections according to your group and its needs. At the end of the planning stage, you will have a set of broad aims, each with a series of objectives that describe how you will achieve your aim and a second set of objectives that set out the specific activities that will be undertaken by the group.

DISCOVERING YOUR CLIENTS' NEEDS AND WANTS

It is relatively easy to work out what you would like to achieve from your classes. It is not always so simple to find out what your client's expectations and needs are, and what they hope to get from attending a group or consultation with you. When asked directly, many pregnant parents will state they don't know what they want from a class. Private consultations are easier in this respect, because these are usually initiated by the client, who will probably know why they are seeing you and what they hope to achieve.

First time parents in particular are often unsure about what they need to know or the purpose of attending a group or class. Perhaps they have joined the group because they think it is the right thing to do, or because they have been told to attend, and so they arrive with very few goals, other than to learn 'everything' about having a baby. As they begin participating in the group, you can arouse their curiosity, inspire them to seek further information and enable them to take responsibility for their own learning. As this happens, group members will begin expressing new needs and these can be incorpo-rated into your objectives.

Many expectant parents have unconscious needs and expectations that affect their participation in the class. Offering an opportunity to explore these in a supportive and safe environment may open up new avenues for discussion and learning and add to the list of objectives for both you and the members of your group. Suggestions for suitable activities to initiate this process are described in Part 3.

OUTCOMES

Outcomes describe the eventual results of an experience, or what happened in the end. Learning outcomes describe the information retained by the learner, or the skills that can be demonstrated by the learner as the result of the instruction they have received. The final result of the learning process can be affected by various factors, some of which are beyond your control as an edu-cator.

For example, a pregnant woman may be able to show you she can correctly position a baby doll as though she was breastfeeding, but by the time the baby is born she may have forgotten the details, due to the length of time since she learned the technique in class. Your objective in having her demonstrate her breastfeeding knowledge using the doll may have been met by her role play, but the learning outcome may not be as good as you hoped. The uncontrolla-ble factor is her memory, which may be affected by the pregnancy hormones.

In an educational sense, learning outcomes must be demonstrable at the end of the class series. If you can show that your class members, at that point, have the skills and information they require, and that your educational objectives have been met, then you have completed your task. It is not wise to use birth outcomes or later parenting behaviours as a measure of your success as an educator, since these will inevitably be affected by a host of factors over which you, and perhaps the parents themselves, have little or no control.

Perhaps the best outcome is for parents to feel satisfied with the way in which they have handled the events surrounding birth and are managing their parenting experiences. Satisfaction is difficult to measure, but it generally includes positive feelings of competence, confidence and skill. A childbirth educator can check that parents have these skills to some extent through par-ticipation in carefully designed activities that show their abilities, but whether parents apply the skills in the event and feel satisfaction as a result, is unpre-dictable. Let's hope that they do!

In summary

- Prepare your global aims for the series of classes as a whole.
- List broad aims for each class within the series.
- Prepare objectives for each global and class aim stating the learning outcome desired for your clients.
- List learner objectives for each topic to be covered — what do your want them to gain from this topic?
- Prepare objectives for each topic that describe various teaching and presentation strategies that will take account of different styles of learning within your group.
- List objectives that will enable you to present the classes (housekeeping).
- List objectives that will help you meet your own needs as an educator.

Further reading

Mager R. 1990, *Preparing Instructional Objectives*, Kogan Page.

Nichols F. H. & Humenick S. 1988, *Childbirth Education: Practice, Research and Theory*, Saunders International.

Wilson P. 1990, *Antenatal Teaching, A guide to theory and practice*, Faber & Faber, London.

Wilberg G. 1992, *Preparing for Birth and Parenthood: awareness training and teaching manual for childbirth professionals*, Butterworths.

CHAPTER 2

HOW ADULTS LEARN

Whenever we take on the role of an educator, we must remind ourselves that people learn in different ways. The majority of those we work with will be adults, who have developed their own pattern for absorbing and assimilating information. Most will also have experience, sometimes considerable, of the educational process, usually acquired from school and perhaps further studies. This previous experience will influence the way they approach their prenatal education. Their attitude to learning, motivation, reason for attending and even what they expect to achieve may all be coloured by the way they have learned or been taught in the past.

Amongst the factors that affect the ease with which people learn are:

- the way in which the information is presented or taught,
- the emotional state of the learner at the time,
- the emotional 'baggage' from earlier life experiences being carried by the learner,
- their readiness for learning at the time,
- what they already know about the subject,
- their general educational level,
- the opportunities to practise or use the new knowledge,
- the feedback they receive from the teacher,
- their own assessment of how useful the learning experience has been.

CHARACTERISTICS OF ADULT LEARNERS

Having adult learners in a group learning situation is enjoyable and rewarding. They have usually nominated to join your group and are therefore motivated and willing to learn. They have much to share and the maturity to benefit from group participation. Whilst they all have their own views, beliefs and responses as individuals, the general characteristics of adults suggest that learning opportunities will be most successful if they:

- are self directed,
- encourage the learner to take responsibility,

- fit comfortably with prior experience,
- are integrated with the learner's beliefs and values, especially those based in culture,
- encourage the use of personal resources,
- encourage group participation and use of group resources,
- meet the learner's needs as well as wants,
- have a stated purpose and a measurable result.

STYLES OF LEARNING

People use their eyes, ears and senses to learn. By the time they have reached adulthood, they have often developed a preference, usually unconscious, for using one or more of these modes when they are learning. In your group, you will be working with people who may learn in different ways. You will have those who primarily use their eyes to receive new information, others who prefer listening, and some who like to get totally involved and use all their senses when learning new skills. Therefore, when presenting your information and devising group activities, you will need to present in various ways to ensure that everyone receives your message.

When learning a practical skill, not only do all the senses need to be involved, but feedback and evaluation through practice is needed (trial and error!) to help cement the new skill into the repertoire, and assist the development of some competence.

All learning requires a measure of practice and feedback, even when the task is to acquire facts, and innate skills such as dexterity may also affect the learning outcome.

The main styles of learning can be classified as visual, auditory or kinaesthetic. Visual learners use their eyes as the primary avenue for learning, auditory learners prefer to use their ears, and kinaesthetic learners like to involve their whole bodies and all their senses as they learn (these people are sometimes described as experiential learners — learning through doing and practical involvement).

VISUAL LEARNING STYLES

Visually oriented people relate comfortably to pictures, demonstrations, models, videos and written material. They also like using their imagination to create mental pictures. This kind of learner is easily recognised — notice the way they brighten up and focus eagerly on charts or the diagram you have drawn on the board. They also comment on the detail in videos, and enjoy reading books and background notes. During discussion they will often use 'visual' words in their responses, such as:

* 'I see what you mean'
* 'It looks like you want me to . . .'
* 'It appears that . . .'
* 'Read my lips!'

You will notice that visual people often stare intently at you when you are speaking, even perhaps frowning as they concentrate with their eyes. Frowning, in this case, may not mean that they don't understand, and you will know this from their feedback.

An example of a visual person is someone who can readily assemble 'do-it-yourself' furniture from a diagram, or a person who enjoys creating models from kits. They are also good at jigsaw puzzles, and can imagine how a house will look just from viewing the plans.

PRESENTING TO VISUAL LEARNERS

It is easy to devise teaching methods for visual learners. Include charts, videos, written material, demonstrations and models. Writing activities, such as taking notes, brainstorming ideas onto butcher's paper, filling in questionnaires, using worksheets and pencil and paper games will all have appeal. Visual learners like to have written reference notes or background reading material to take home. They will appreciate metaphors and mental imagery, and can 'picture' themselves in various situations.

Remember, however, that just because someone is a visual learner, it doesn't mean that they are not also listening to what you are saying — they are just preferentially absorbing your message using their eyes.

Your own behaviour should include: little physical movement (try not to walk around or move a lot as this will be distracting), facing them when talking so they can see your mouth, and the use of examples and statistics. Allow for thinking time in the group when they may be making mental pictures in response to your question or presentation of facts.

AUDITORY LEARNERS

People who are 'auditory' learners use their sense of hearing as a primary means of absorbing information. They enjoy verbal involvement, and the use of sound or aural cues as part of the teaching/learning process. Auditory learners like discussion, hearing of other's experiences and story telling. They are comfortable with verbal instructions and can follow spoken descriptions.

In your group, you may be able to identify these people from their behaviour — they tend to look down or close their eyes as they listen intently, as eye contact is not so important for these learners. Don't think they are asleep!

An example of an auditory learner is someone who can pick up a new language from listening to a set of spoken word tapes. They enjoy radio programs, notice the sound track on a video or film, and like music and singing.

Auditory learners can be identified by the way they like to talk things over and debate issues, and also from their conversation, which often includes clues to their learning orientation:

- 'Sounds as if you'd like me to . . .'
- 'I hear what you are saying'
- 'Tell me about it again'
- 'Listen to me!'

PRESENTING TO AUDITORY LEARNERS

This group likes discussion — in small groups, large groups or individually. They like hearing stories, listening to audiotapes (sounds of labour, new babies, etc.) and will enjoy videos. They like music and verbal memory cues (remember 'a relaxed jaw is a relaxed perineum'?). Because they are tuned in to sound, be aware of background noises or chatter in the group, which will tend to distract this kind of learner.

Your behaviour should include: having them repeat information when answering questions, arranging your material in a sequence that is covered step by step, and interaction with individuals.

KINAESTHETIC LEARNERS

People who prefer kinaesthetic learning opportunities will be seeking activities that engage all their senses and involve their whole body. They will benefit from practical sessions and like activities that use physical movement, such as role plays, exercise sessions, labour ward tours and demonstrations. They also like using their imagination, and tapping into their emotions and feelings. They like touch and feel comfortable in practical sessions such as labour rehearsals. You will notice them drumming their fingers, nodding their heads, wiggling their feet or generally fiddling, and they often gesticulate or move around when they are talking.

This kind of learner can be identified by their language too:

- 'I get the feeling that . . .'
- 'I wonder if I could . . .'

- 'I sense that . . .'
- 'I don't get the point of . . .'

PRESENTING TO KINAESTHETIC LEARNERS

Devise teaching strategies that include exercise sessions, massage, practice of positions for labour, holding new babies, handling models, role plays. Involve them as much as possible and avoid sessions with a lot of sitting.

Your own behaviour should include: moving around, some 'acting', use of a wide vocabulary, discussion on emotions and feelings, talking slowly and standing close and even touching, when appropriate.

INVOLVING ALL THREE

Although most adults will have a preferred learning style, everyone tends to use more than one, and possibly all three on occasion. Just because someone is predominantly visually oriented doesn't mean that they can't understand verbal instructions or might not benefit from practical experience. When learning a new skill, such as changing a nappy, it may take all three — looking at a set of instructional pictures, having someone telling you what to do, and actually practising it on the baby. Since becoming a parent involves acquiring or developing a number of skills, a multi-sensual approach in your teaching will offer the best chance of successfully reaching everyone in your group. With important themes or facts, consider offering them in at least three different ways to increase the likelihood of your message getting through.

Many people, in the end, gain most from experience. Indeed, some skills, such as learning to drive a car, can only be learned through practice, even when a new driver has a thorough understanding of the road rules! Becoming a parent for the first time is another example, where knowing the theory, reading the books, listening to other parents' stories and seeing examples of parenting behaviour all around them are poor substitutes for 'hands-on' experience.

In any group of learners there will be a mixture of learning styles, so it will be important to include activities that will appeal to everyone. Your first session should incorporate presentations in all three learning styles so that everyone in the group feels included. Early success with learning something new encourages participants to come back for more and boosts confidence. It is also empowering to feel that one has successfully gained a skill which can then be used when needed. The skill may be a new way to talk to the doctor or a self-help idea for easing labour pain — the important thing is to know you have it when you need it!

As the group develops, you will begin to notice some of the characteristics of the differing learning styles and if you sense that the majority have one pre-

TABLE 2: *Characteristics of visual, auditory and kinaesthetic learners.*

	Visual	Auditory	Kinaesthetic
Eyes	Glance upwards in response, lift eyes when thinking.	Glance sideways when responding or thinking.	Glance down, drop eyes when thinking or before responding.
Body movement	Sit and concentrate, stare ahead, frown.	Rhythmical movements. Close eyes to listen intently.	Restless, shifts whole body, fiddles, doodles, gesticulates with hands when speaking.
Words used in speech	See, looks like, appears, focus, clear, picture, notice.	Sounds like, I hear, tell me, listen, said, talk.	Feels like, grasp, action words (run through, hold it), sense, wonder.
Presenter style	Sit or stand straight and still. Speak rapidly. Focus on visual aids.	Variation in voice pitch, volume, speed, tone. Rhythmic movements, discussion, music, catchy phrases, interaction.	Link different gestures to specific content. Exaggeration, emphasis, full descriptions. Involvement in participatory learning.

dominant style, you can gear many of your teaching strategies accordingly. As a general rule, however, plan to present your material in at least three different ways so that your message is reinforced, there is variety in your teaching and so your group members are more likely to understand the content.

When working with an individual, it is usually easier to determine the learning style, since you can concentrate on just one set of responses. In some situations, such as talking to a person on the telephone, you will need to rely on their language to give you clues, since you can't evaluate their reactions in person. When you are giving information to just one person, use their preferred style if you can, most of the time, but do include the other senses too, to broaden the learning opportunity.

While experiential learning will probably be very effective for adult learners, it will not suit everyone. Some people like participating, experimenting and being involved in the games and activities. Others prefer to just sit and watch, learning through observation while deciding on their own course of action privately. Some people prefer to listen and look, and to think about their own choices without necessarily sharing with others. Many like to have a skill or technique demonstrated before they try it out themselves. They will participate, but only after being shown what to do first. These are all variations on learning styles that are quite common among adults. Try and accommodate all of these preferences by allowing the group members to choose their own degree of participation.

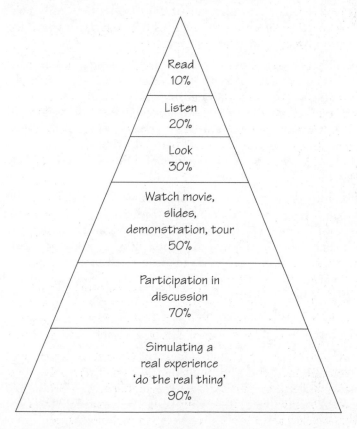

FIGURE 1: *Likely retention rates for adults for different methods of learning.*

OTHER LEARNING STATES

Once information has been received by an adult learner, they then go through other steps to assimilate and organise the information ready for later use. There are many ways people arrange and store facts in their memories, and being aware of some common approaches will help you to refine your teaching presentations.

THE INFORMATION JIGSAW

Some people find it easier to piece together the full story from a series of smaller facts which they arrange and fit together to arrive at a coherent overall picture. Others like to start with an overview of the whole, then break it into smaller pieces to explore in depth, knowing where each one fits into the broad scheme. Either way, it is important for a learner to have both a sense of the big picture as well as an appreciation of all the fragments from which it is composed. Whether a learner progresses from small to large or from large to small will be a matter of personal preference.

It is essential that an educator can identify both the big picture and the smaller components for each of the topics or themes in the class series. To take account of both learning styles described here, try introducing your topic using the 'big picture' (an overview), then break it down into smaller segments and deal with those in turn, and then summarise, placing the smaller pieces into the broader view to outline the big picture again. By doing this you will help both styles of learner see how it all fits together, and they will have a more coherent grasp of the topic.

To enhance your presentation, try using a visual representation, by drawing diagrams to illustrate both the macro and micro positions. Having a visual reference point will help the group to stay focused, and to make sense of complex topics. For example, using a diagram of the 'cascade of intervention' in the birth process makes it easier to see how each intervention is either the result of, or precipitates, another intervention. It also makes it easier to see where an individual intervention, such as induction, or epidural fits in relation to the whole intervention process.

LINEAR AND LATERAL LEARNERS

A linear learner takes a series of steps in sequence in order to learn effectively. For them, each piece of information needs to build on what has gone before, in logical progression. It is a neat and tidy approach, and one which is fostered in school. This orderly approach makes learning easy, through a series of clearly identified steps based on an assumption of predictable outcomes at

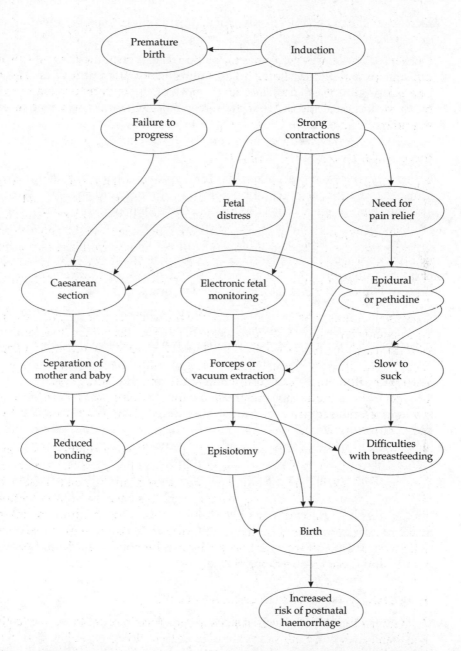

FIGURE 2: *The big picture showing the "cascade of intervention" in birth following an induction. Each box represents a micro topic within the macro or big picture.*

each stage. It can be very effective for acquiring skills that lend themselves to this approach, such as learning a new language, or learning to cook.

These kinds of learners may have trouble when working with events which are not predictable or capable of being organised. Parenting and the birth process offer appropriate examples. In both of these cases, learning is often haphazard as the unpredictable takes over. Since outcomes are never assured, much flexibility is needed and if a parent needs a logical progression to their learning, they may feel unable to cope with the chaotic sequence of events, and unskilled as a result.

Lateral learners have quite a different approach. They are able to take a number of haphazard facts, find common threads and then, if necessary, arrange them in a linear way to demonstrate their understanding. For this kind of learner, making order out of chaos is easy, and they are comfortable moving from one topic or another in an apparently disconnected way. Linear learners may need to complete all the border of a jigsaw puzzle before they fill in the middle, whereas a lateral learner may work on smaller segments at random, only piecing it all together and completing the border at the end.

In many ways, lateral learners find it easier to make sense of the unpredictability of labour, birth and parenting. Linear learners will need help to see their progress in learning the necessary skills and to feel they are capable of dealing with unexpected events.

The childbirth educator can provide useful role modelling, particularly by demonstrating that it is possible to deviate from a structured format or sequence of class topics and deal with random questions while still keeping the group on an overall track. This may not be easy at first, but is an important skill that will be developed through experience. It is also an example of the conflict that can occur between *needs* and *wants*: as an educator we often need to feel organised, with a coherent, demonstrable structure for our teaching and presentation. On the other hand, we want to appear flexible, able to manage the unexpected and willing to put our clients needs before our own.

Similarly, our group members may want to have all the information presented to them neatly in an organised fashion, but may need to see that the life events of birth and parenting are unpredictable, even chaotic, in nature.

NOTE YOUR OWN STYLE!

Just as the members of your group are all experienced adult learners with their own preferred style, you too have a background that will have influenced the way you learn and teach. Your natural tendency will be to present your material as you would like to receive it yourself in a learning situation. You will be most comfortable using behaviours that are typical of your preferred learning style, since these are what you have recognised and modelled from others.

If, however, you present constantly in, for example, a visual style, and your group are mostly auditory learners, there is a risk that they will not hear what they need, and that they may miss important information. It will be helpful for you to analyse your teaching methods. You could try:

- Tape recording a group or class and analysing your presentation for visual, auditory and kinaesthetic words that you have used.
- Videotaping and observing your own patterns of behaviour when presenting. Where do you look? Do you move around? What do you do with your hands? Again, does your language indicate your own visual, auditory or kinaesthetic preference?
- Writing an account of an event and checking out the language.
- Imagining you are teaching someone who is deaf or blind.
- Changing your own style, by substituting auditory for visual words, etc., in your written account.

Are you a linear or lateral learner yourself? This will also influence your teaching style, and how comfortable you feel while teaching. You may be stressed by constant interruptions or stray questions if you prefer to be organised and logical with your presentation, and this may be a reflection of your own approach to learning.

Do you prefer to work from the big picture to the detail or the other way around? Identifying your own preference in this area will help you to compensate so you can better serve your client's learning needs.

Once you are aware of your own preferred learning styles, you can actively modify your teaching to allow for the learning styles of other people. This will become easier as you become more confident with the specific content of your classes. In time, your familiarity with the information will allow you to concentrate on the *way* you say something, your posture, your use of teaching aids, your selection of educational activities and so on. Watching experienced childbirth educators at work will help you see this in action. Don't be discouraged by their seemingly effortless group and teaching skills — they have only arrived at this degree of competence through practice and constant evaluation. You will get there in time too!

READINESS FOR LEARNING

It seems self evident that acquiring information or learning a skill is easier when the time and conditions are right for the learner. If you are not sure if the learner is ready, you will need to arouse interest in the topic first, and judge their reaction. This could be done by using an agenda setting exercise, for example. Alternatively, you can note the questions being raised, as they will indicate that the time is right for discussion on a topic. Having receptive learners in your group will make all the difference.

Most adults will remember times when they struggled to grasp some new concept or learn important facts, only to feel unhappy or even demoralised by a perceived inability to learn. Many factors can contribute to this lack of success: being forced to learn something when it is not of interest; poor teaching; personal problems that interfere with concentration; difficult physical surroundings etc.

Similarly, most people can remember, often with pleasure, skills or information acquired easily, as a result of positive circumstances and good teaching.

Even when people are eager to learn, and the educational environment is positive, the learning outcome can be hampered by factors that are not within their personal control or by unexpected events that occur. If there are no opportunities to put the new skills to use immediately or to test the newly acquired knowledge in a practical way, the impetus is lost and the new information forgotten.

Most expectant parents come to classes with a very positive attitude towards gaining information. Even those who are reluctant at first can often be encouraged to learn practical skills if the educator uses motivational methods in presenting class material.

However, even the keenest group member may have difficulty absorbing information if it is presented at a time when it seems personally irrelevant or inappropriate. Many childbirth educators will recall comments made by parents at post-natal reunions that not enough attention was paid to babycare topics, or the emotional upheaval a new baby can elicit in inexperienced parents. 'You never told me it would be like this!' is a common wail heard at these gatherings. In reality, the educator may have allocated a significant proportion of class time to parenting issues. Much attention may have been given to detail, and a number of interesting strategies used to convey both the practicalities and emotional aspects of babycare in the early weeks after birth. Why do some people fail to absorb this information or forget that it was even covered? There are many possible reasons, and discovering these forms an important part of the evaluation process. Leaving aside teaching strategies and presentation methods for the moment (although these need to be critically analysed as well) let us consider the issue of readiness for learning. Asking these questions may reveal useful insights:

- At what stage in the pregnancy was the parenting information offered to parents?
- Were they ready to look at post-natal issues?
- Was the information tacked on at the end of class series, following on from birth topics?
- Was there enough time given to parenting topics, or were some abbreviated or eliminated due to time constraints?
- Were the participants more focused on the labour and birth at the time the information was covered?
- Were practical topics, such as breastfeeding, bathing and nappy changing able to be reinforced through practical sessions with real babies, soon after the demonstration?

And finally,

- If you were pregnant, when would you find it useful to discuss parenting issues?
- At what stage of your pregnancy would you be interested in these topics?

In reviewing the answers to these questions, it can be noted that parenting topics can be loosely divided into two main areas: practical skills and emotional/psychological issues surrounding the new status of parenthood. If, from an educational standpoint, the most appropriate time to schedule discussion is when expectant parents are ready to absorb and use the information, then it becomes apparent that re-organising the class sessions to offer the information when it is most needed will be more successful.

Emotional and psychological issues need exploration during the early part of pregnancy, when parents are discovering the joys and disruptions of lifestyle and relationship changes brought about by the pregnancy. An appropriate time would be around 24–28 weeks, when the baby is making its presence felt and parents are planning domestic arrangements for accommodating and caring for the new family member. The birth itself is far enough away not to be of immediate concern, and parents are facing a number of changes that can be addressed in a class group. Scheduling parenting in one or more separate classes or sessions emphasises the importance of these issues and allows them to be explored at an appropriate time, without the impending birth creating a distraction. Breaking up the traditional 7 or 8 week series into sections covering early pregnancy, parenting and birth also allows the group to meet over an extended period of time, which fosters social contact and helps the group to 'grow' together.

Babycare skills become an urgent necessity when a new mother is confronted with a dirty nappy or a hungry baby within hours of the birth. No amount of practice with a doll can ever simulate the realities of trying to attach a nappy to a squirming newborn, and no amount of tucking a doll against a pregnant breast will reveal the intricacies of feeding a hungry baby. Perhaps the most appropriate time for learning about newborn care is when it is most needed, that is, in the post-natal period. Programs where mothers are helped to learn necessary skills, with their own baby during the post-natal period, would seem to have the greatest potential for success. Positive reinforcement, praise and use of self directed learning will be important factors in empowering mothers at this sensitive time. The potential for improved self-esteem and confidence in mothers is almost limitless, providing that the educator (who will probably be the midwife on the post-natal ward) is aware of basic educational techniques for fostering these attributes in new mothers.

Parenting topics form just one example where appropriate timing of the information and practical sessions may be critical to successful learning. Consider all the topics you have scheduled for your classes. When is it likely that expectant parents would be ready for these discussions? Topics you may like to consider carefully in this regard are: nutrition, pregnancy fitness and exercise, pregnancy discomforts, pre-natal screening and diagnosis, premature labour, choosing birthplace and caregivers, breastfeeding, contraception and emotional and physical adjustment. In fact — all your class topics should be included in this list!

LANGUAGE

What we say and the words we use are the very essence of communication. When teaching, there are several aspects of language usage that we must consider. This means thinking not only about the specific words we choose — we must also include their interpretation by the listener, the connotations they suggest and the way in which they are uttered. The non-verbal behaviour that accompanies our speech also has an important effect on the way our words are received.

The written language of birth has evolved over several centuries. The midwives who traditionally cared for women during childbearing before doctors became involved were largely illiterate, and probably had specific spoken language to describe pregnancy and birth, based on women's perceptions of these events. When doctors developed obstetrics as a speciality they described pregnancy and birth using medical terminology, imposing in the process a peculiarly negative connotation for these normal bodily functions.

This legacy of largely negative medical terms and descriptions for essentially natural events is now so commonly accepted that little attention is paid by health professionals to the impact of this language on the pregnant women — we hardly notice what we are saying!

The problem with these medical terms and descriptions is that they convey a specific view of the process, usually negative or doubtful, in contrast to the reality that pregnancy and birth are normal circumstances for women nearly all the time. Today, we find ourselves in the ludicrous situation of having to use technical and medical terminology to describe natural processes since there are no acceptable 'feminine' substitutes. We use words like 'confinement' and 'delivery' when we really mean 'labour' and 'giving birth', and this has become so commonplace that it takes conscious effort to reshape our thinking through the use of more appropriate language. Even the word 'mother' has come to be debased in our culture and contains a fairly negative put-down in our materialistic, career oriented society. In order to regain some status for our mothers we may have to resort to using 'women' (e.g. pregnant women, women with new babies etc.) to remind caregivers that these are real people, worthy of consideration!

There can be no doubt that the words we use reinforce our notions of the events or situations we are describing. Perhaps it is no accident that so much of the vocabulary in use in obstetrics is negative, masculine, dominating and anti-woman. Men will never have insights on birth drawn from personal experience — they will always have to form their views of the process from the position of an observer, not a participant, and at times it must look rather threatening and traumatic. In addition, the medical model of needing to help, or rescue a woman in apparent distress during labour will inevitably mean the introduction of medical terms to describe the 'treatments' being used.

The pregnant women with whom we work are coerced into adopting this medical view of their physical state every time medical terms are used by their caregivers. This, of course, may be an unconscious or even deliberate part of the agenda: the sooner the pregnant woman learns to accept the medical viewpoint, the easier it will be to gain her compliance and to focus her natural dependency during pregnancy onto professional carers. Reinforcing the idea that pregnancy and birth are complicated and mysterious processes, only really understood by the 'experts', is also part of this agenda. Given the insidious and pervasive nature of the masculine, medical and negative language in use today in midwifery and obstetrics, is will be hard for women to feel empowered and confident as they explore the natural wonders of pregnancy and birth. Perhaps one of the most important services we could offer women during pre-natal classes is to help them develop a new vocabulary for childbearing, based on a feminine, midwifery oriented perspective of these events.

As an educator, you can have a major influence on the way women view birth. But first, be aware of the language you are using in your communications! Consider these alternatives to commonly used words and phrases:

Usually used	Try instead
fetus	baby
contractions (of the uterus)	expansions (of the cervix)
caesarean section	caesarean birth
labour	birth process, journey (as appropriate)
delivery	birth
antenatal	pre-natal
class	group, session, discussion
coping (with labour, pain etc.)	managing (labour, pain etc.)
birth plan	guidelines for birth

There are also some downright negative phrases and terms which should be removed from our vocabularies:

Usually used	Try instead
adequate pelvis	capable pelvis
failure to progress	pause in labour
expected date of confinement	approximate birth date
incompetent cervix	elastic cervix
girls, ladies	women
trial of labour	vaginal birth after previous caesarean birth
control (of anything) during labour	delete — birth is uncontrollable
losing (lost) a baby	the baby died

In addition to the specific words we use, we must also be aware that the way in which they are said will have an impact on the recipient. Many words carry emotional implications for some people, perhaps because of their experiences or because of a more general connotation. For example, pregnant women hearing the word 'forceps' may feel frightened or anxious, since for some people this word conjures up images of complications or emergencies, especially for the baby. Personal experience may play a part — a woman whose baby was born using forceps may react to this word either positively or negatively depending on her perception of the events surrounding the birth and her emotional state at the time. Many people will react to certain words or phrases used to describe birth, as revealed by their unconscious and conscious reactions to this word used in conversation. Noting this reaction can be helpful for an educator who is trying to assess the potential fears and anxieties in her clients.

Since we have a goal of helping women develop positive views on their ability to give birth, we must be aware of hidden traps in the language we use. People's perceptions of our words are not predictable therefore we must be vigilant for unexpected negative reactions to what we are saying. Personal experiences, attitudes, feelings and knowledge levels will shape the way people interpret words and we should be ready to accept that other people, especially the sensitive pregnant woman, may receive our message in quite a different way from our intention.

Voice speed, tone, inflexions and emphasis add colour to our language as well. The impact of a word can be altered dramatically through emphasis or tone, and the speed at which we speak also affects its reception. Try audiotaping a segment of your class, perhaps an information session on a topic with the potential for emotional reactions (e.g. drugs in labour, or complications during birth). Analyse your words, note your tone, speed and emphasis and listen for the reactions in your group. Would changing your language or altering your delivery make a difference to the way your speech was received by your group?

One last point on spoken language: repetition can be a useful tool in your teaching. Positive phrases, positive pieces of information, carefully chosen words, that are used repeatedly have the potential to become anchored in the subconscious thinking of the recipient. Another way of looking at this phenomenon is to remember that if you say something often enough there is a tendency to start believing it! Affirmations are based on this principle, but the effect can be broadened to include other basic messages or snippets of key information that would be beneficial for women. An oft repeated message, delivered in a variety of ways at different times throughout a series of meetings can have the same effect. Examples are 'trust your body to let you know what you need to do in labour', 'all kinds of emotional reactions to these events are possible', 'be guided by your baby's needs during the first months after birth' etc.

NON-VERBAL BEHAVIOUR

Communication is more than just speaking — it involves messages sent via non-verbal cues as well, and these are just as important as the words being used. The non-verbal component of our communications includes all the various postures, facial expressions, arm actions, body movements etc. that accompany our voice. Much of the subconscious message gets through via this 'body language' and the impression we make by the way we look is sometimes more powerful than what we are saying.

When we meet someone for the first time, we often form an instant opinion about that person, long before they have spoken. We take our cues from their appearance, their stance, the look on their face, their body actions — all kinds of small clues are pieced together to help us form our impression of the person. It takes place so fast, and so unconsciously that we can sometimes be surprised that when we do begin conversation, we discover that our first impression can either be confirmed or is unsupported. Changing a first impression can be difficult: it is as if we have to consciously override the unconscious conclusions we have instantly formed through our interpretation of the person's non-verbal behaviours. Can you remember an occasion when you formed a view of someone at a distance, only to discover on meeting them that they were quite different from what you had imagined? Do you remember the surprise surrounding this discovery, and how it took conscious recognition that you had perhaps formed a hasty decision about the person?

The non-verbal message that accompanies spoken words has a powerful effect on the recipient. Imagine how you would feel if, when he was taking your blood pressure, the doctor raised his left eyebrow a fraction. What would you tend to think? Would you necessarily guess that he was hard of hearing, or would you jump to a conclusion that you had a blood pressure problem?

It is important that non-verbal behaviour matches the spoken word appropriately. For example, serious topics will be best received if accompanied by a serious tone of voice, quiet, restrained body movements and a 'straight' facial expression. Lighter topics can be delivered with smiles, even laughter, hand movement, body action and variable voice tones. Much of this is automatic during communication, but non-verbals can unconsciously reflect the attitude and values of the presenter. If these unconsciously expressed values and attitudes match those of the recipient, the message will be clear: we both feel the same way about this topic. If, however, the recipient has a different attitude towards a subject, then he may feel out of step with the presenter, or that they are on different wavelengths. Similarly, if the presenter uses inappropriate non-verbal behaviour to accompany a spoken message, confusion can arise in the recipient: what is actually being said? The voice is saying one thing but there is quite a different message being registered at the same time from the unspoken body actions. Which is to be believed? The influence of non-verbal behaviour on the impact of a message can be quite profound.

Checking out your presentation style through using videotape feedback will help you make sure that your non-verbal behaviours are appropriate, that they are not confusing group members, and that they are not influencing others through conveying messages about your own attitudes and values.

You can also use the power of non-verbal communication to enhance your presentation. Try livening up the discussion by raising your voice or increasing its tone and volume. Moving your position, perhaps standing up, will attract attention and shift the focus back to you as a leader. If the energy levels are falling, change activities to brighten up the group, and choose one that involves moving around.

A group generally reflects (mirrors) the mood and style of the leader. If you are quiet and reserved, they will tend to copy this behaviour. Energetic and outgoing leaders tend to have groups where members are more likely to speak up and enjoy participation. If you are feeling emotionally flat, tired, or lacking in energy, your group will tend to reflect this. We all have times when we are not feeling our best when we are teaching, so try to be aware of these occasions so you can avoid unhelpful non-verbal indicators of your feelings that will inhibit the group's responses.

Using the group's experience

The group process is of primary importance to the success of pre-natal education. Your clients meet as a group, share individual and collective experiences of pregnancy, form social bonds and work towards common goals. One of your tasks, as leader of this group, is to facilitate this process and to make every effort to ensure that the benefits of group work are available for the participants.

Learning about group dynamics and functioning is beyond the scope of this book. However, there are many excellent resources available, and a selection of these is listed at the end of this chapter.

In the context of empowerment, learning from others, especially in a group setting, can be an important factor for many women. Pregnancy is a time for sharing stories, listening to others' experiences, and noticing the effects of the emotional and psychological impact of birth and new parenthood on friends. Many pregnant women become the recipients of 'horror' stories and tales of woe, and if a woman hears enough of these, she may begin to believe that these experiences are universal, which can be negative and undermine her confidence. Women who have positive stories to tell of normal births often say little in a negative climate, perhaps because they have no grief to relieve.

Speaking out against the common experience also sets one apart in the broad group and puts further pressure on those still suffering.

Being part of a pre-natal group whose focus is positive and empowering may help women to see these issues more clearly. If the stories they are hearing elsewhere have negative connotations, positive inputs will be necessary to make sure that pregnant women get a balanced view. With this need in mind, an educator or group leader can plan specific activities where these issues can be explored. The group setting is an ideal medium for this to occur. In the same way, cultural attitudes and behaviours, expectations of caregivers, family dynamics and other broad issues can be usefully explored. These kinds of discussions help to put birth in our society into perspective, and may assist group members to understand the values placed on birth. For example, encouraging the group to discuss why women give birth lying down can lead to interesting insights into the broad political climate that operates in our hospitals. This kind of discussion often arises after the group have been discovering the unique design of the pelvis and the way it functions in labour. As a leader, all you need do is facilitate group exploration of the issues. When a woman realises the politics of supine birth, she is much better equipped to devise appropriate alternatives!

Using group experiences as a basis for your teaching can be useful in other ways as well. It is likely that everyone in your group already has considerable knowledge, information and even practical experience of parenthood that can be utilised in your teaching.

Firstly, everyone was a child once, and this will have bestowed a legacy of parenting styles and strategies that will influence behaviours and beliefs in the adult. These often come into sharper focus when the adult is evaluating possible parenting behaviours for themselves!

Secondly, most adults know something about pregnancy and birth — information gleaned from a variety of sources over the years. Much of this surfaces when a pregnancy occurs, and forms a foundation for further information, which prospective parents seek everywhere.

Therefore, everyone in your group is likely to know something about being pregnant, the birth process and babycare issues, before you begin the classes. The information they have may not be complete, or accurate, but one reason they have joined the class may be to fill in the gaps. It is important, in the empowerment process, to validate and acknowledge the information that people already have, since this is one way of confirming that expectant parents already have considerable skills and know-how, ready to be applied to their coming parenting experiences. Of course, you may have to gently correct misinformation, but recognising that parents-to-be are already quite knowledgeable can be reassuring and boost confidence levels (yours and theirs) considerably.

You can use this pre-existing knowledge most effectively when setting agendas and negotiating class formats with your group. You will save much teaching time if you establish what is already known, and work on from there to flesh out the basics with additional material as requested by the group.

When people share what they already know, in a group setting, they are using the opportunity to learn from each other. It has sometimes been said that it is possible for all the information needed by new parents to be already present within the group, with each person having part of the story. The group leader's role in this situation is to make sure that everyone shares their information to build up a full picture for each individual. The advantage of this approach is that your role becomes that of a facilitator rather than an 'expert' source of information, and you can adjust your presentation style from being a teacher to being a group leader. It will also help you develop your counselling skills.

While using group resources is generally helpful to individuals and leaders, there are some occasions when this approach must be treated with caution. In classes where experienced parents are mixed with those expecting their first baby, situations can arise where the experienced ones either dominate the group or are exploited by the leader to teach the others. Parents coming to class in order to refresh their labour and birth knowledge sometimes need to debrief their past experiences, and this can turn into a frightening series of 'horror' stories which alarms and unnerves the rest of the group. You will need to be prepared for this outcome with some strategies for turning these negative experiences into positive plans for action, and for dealing with the feelings generated by these stories. Since this kind of event can't be predicted, you could consider seeing all your refresher parents in a special group of their own, which will avoid them unintentionally influencing prospective first-time parents negatively.

Another problem in using the group's resources can occur when myths or misinformation are accidentally perpetuated. This can happen if, for example, a small group is asked to explore a topic that is unfamiliar. Imagine that a small group is asked to list the advantages and disadvantages of epidurals when they know little about the subject and have not had basic information presented to them in advance. It is possible that various myths and incorrect facts will be discussed if people just draw on what they have heard, and since this conversation is happening in a small group, you, as the leader, may have no input into the discussion. A result could be that 'the blind lead the blind' and unhelpful or even dangerous information is reinforced in people's minds.

Careful planning and selection of appropriate discussion topics and activities will help you to avoid this situation.

It is also possible to exploit the resources of class couples by using techniques such as setting 'homework' or research projects for them to complete between classes. As a health professional, it is your responsibility to give them the basic information they need as part of the service. If people want to explore a subject in more depth, then they can be shown where to find additional information, or be given material to read. Setting 'homework' is also reminiscent of school, which many people would not rank among the best learning experiences of their lives.

Learning from each other is a natural process, and modelling the behaviour of others is a primary educational tool. Children learn much by copying, as parents discover to their surprise and delight, and applying this strategy with adults can be useful in class. Role play, problem solving activities and participation in practical exercises all draw on this mode of learning. Working within a group can enhance modelling behaviours as people share reactions, explore various emotions, devise alternative approaches and discuss the issues surrounding parenting. Having access to a variety of viewpoints, and being able to hear other people's insights is one of the greatest benefits of prenatal classes, and we should make every effort to use these powerful potentials for the benefit of our group.

IN SUMMARY

Working with adults is rewarding and exciting, if you remember that:

- They bring a rich background to your group.
- They like to learn in a variety of ways, that draw on their skills and experience.
- Catering for these different learning styles gives you the chance to develop a wide variety of teaching strategies and presentation ideas, that can make your classes fun as well as informative.
- Every topic can, and should, be taught in at least three different ways (auditory, visual and kinaesthetic) to ensure your message reaches its target.
- Adults like to know where their learning is leading — to see the big picture. Some people need this big picture first, others like to construct it in stages, like a jigsaw.
- Lateral thinking is an important part of problem solving: find ways of encouraging it in your teaching sessions.
- Your own learning style will be reflected in your teaching. Analysing your own presentations is an important step in your professional development.
- People learn best when they are ready and able to learn. Consider issues of relevance, timing and the physical state of your clients.
- Spoken language is central to most communication. Keep your words positive, simple, non-medical and inspiring. Check your voice level, emphasis and intonation too.
- Non-verbal language also conveys powerful messages. What you say with your facial expression and body movements should match your words to convey sincerity and credibility.
- Your class members have much to offer you and the group — recognise their contributions, validate their resources and extend their existing skills.
- Your job is to lead, to empower, to inspire and to support. You don't have to 'teach' them, you just have to help them learn.

FURTHER READING

Enkin M. 1990, 'Commentary: Are the correct outcomes of prenatal education being measured?', *Birth*, vol. 17, no. 2.

Hetherington S. 1990, 'A controlled study of the effect of prepared childbirth classes on obstetric outcome', *Birth*, vol. 17, no. 2.

Knowles M. 1975, *Self Directed Learning*, Cambridge Hall, New Jersey, USA.

Shearer M. 1990, 'Effects of prenatal education depend on the attitudes and practices of obstetric caregivers', *Birth*, vol. 17, no. 2.

Simkin P. & Enkin M. 1989, 'Antenatal classes' in *Effective Care in Pregnancy and Childbirth*, eds I. Chalmers, M. Enkin & M. Keirse, Oxford University Press, Oxford.

CHAPTER 3

THE LEARNING CLIMATE

Just as adults like to have information presented to them in a way they can readily understand, they also need to be in the right frame of mind to receive your message. There are many things that can affect our learning state at any given time. Some of them are physical, such as tiredness, boredom, interest level and comfort, while other factors relate more to our emotional state, such as embarrassment, anxiety, curiosity or our feeling of acceptance within the group. As a group leader, you will need to take care of as many of the negative barriers to learning as you can. Being aware of your group members' emotional and physical states is an important starting point.

PHYSICAL NEEDS

It is much harder to pay attention if your seat is uncomfortable, the room is stuffy or you are desperate to go to the toilet. Pregnant women often find themselves physically uncomfortable and this can make it hard for them to fully participate or absorb information. When you are setting up your group it pays to take care of basic physical needs. You may be very familiar with the room you have chosen for your class, but how would it appear to the members of your group? Try looking at it through their eyes, as if you were pregnant:

- Does it feel welcoming?
- Is there good light and ventilation?
- Is the room warm/cool?
- Does it look cramped and will there be enough space to spread out on the floor for exercises?
- Are there a variety of chairs so each group member can choose something suitable? (Many women find bean bags impossible to get in and out of, and men often find sitting on cushions or mats on the floor very uncomfortable).
- Where are the toilets?
- Are drinks easily accessible?
- Are there distracting charts or equipment that focus attention elsewhere?

- Is there parking nearby, or easy access to public transport?

Having a break in the class format, varying the activities between sitting and participatory exercises and scheduling the class at a suitable hour to avoid fatigue should all be basic to your planning.

You can also invite your group to take some responsibility for their own comfort, just as they will do in labour. They can bring extra pillows, choose seats (and use them) according to their need for comfort or a change of position, and wear suitable clothing for exercising.

If your group starts early in the evening, consider beginning with refreshments, even a substantial snack (perhaps the group could bring their own?) to avoid hunger and an impatience to get home for dinner.

EMOTIONAL AND PSYCHOLOGICAL NEEDS

We all have emotional and psychological needs that influence the way we view the world. A pregnant woman is in a particularly vulnerable emotional and psychological state, and her partner's needs will have changed as well. Pregnancy can be a stressful time for many people as they cope with upheavals in their lifestyle, bodily changes brought on by the growing baby and adjustments to changing roles and added responsibilities. In addition, the pregnant couple have embarked on an extensive voyage of discovery about themselves and the mysteries and magic of becoming parents.

These nine months offer a unique potential for learning a whole range of life skills, some specific to parenting and others of a more general nature. Pregnant women are usually ready and more than willing to learn, so our task as a leader of a pre-natal group should be easy. However, the enormous number of changes going on, the newness of the whole experience and the innate dependency and need for protection and nurturing felt by pregnant women can create a whole range of emotional reactions and heightened psychological needs that can become blocks to effective learning. If we are to tap into the special potential of pregnancy as a time for the learning of life skills, then these specific needs of the individuals in your group must be addressed.

While it is important to try and meet the needs of your group members, there are limitations to what you can reasonably expect to achieve. Pre-natal classes are not group therapy sessions and you are probably not equipped to help people unravel their innermost psychological needs, even if you suspect that these needs are making it hard for someone to learn effectively. You may be concerned that these may interfere with the way a woman will labour or even nurture her child, and often all you can do is suggest some further sources of support or other health professionals who may be better equipped to assist. Having a prepared list of these people that you take with you to the class will enable you to offer an immediate suggestion.

Having recognised that some people have psychological needs that cannot be met by you or your group, it is possible to help many people explore their emotional reactions and your efforts in doing this will be rewarded by increased satisfaction with your teaching within the group and with yourself.

Expectant parents could experience a range of reactions and feelings as they journey through pregnancy and birth. Some of these may be puzzlement, curiosity, anxiety, excitement, fear, concern and confusion. Sharing these feelings with others can enhance the overall experience. Anxieties and worries may be reduced if they are acknowledged, and it may be possible to eliminate some altogether if solutions can be found for problems, or questions can be answered with factual information. This, after all, was the basis of the first pre-natal classes organised by Grantly Dick-Read in Britain during the 1940s. He felt that if adrenalin levels were lowered by reducing fear in labour through better pre-natal education, labour would be shorter and less painful.

So, how can we help people explore fears and anxieties during their pregnancy? There are a number of strategies you can try, but first:

BE AWARE OF YOUR OWN NEEDS

Childbirth educators have their own particular needs, emotions, feelings, fears and anxieties. We also become stressed, upset and challenged from time to time. Sometimes our own physical and emotional state can interfere with our client's opportunities for effective learning, as we are unable to function as well as we would normally, and our group suffers as a result. It may not happen often, but, being only human, we have to recognise that it may happen sometimes. Once we can acknowledge that we may be vulnerable to our own feelings at times, we can prepare some strategies to help ourselves should the situation occur.

As an educator you have certain professional responsibilities, to your client and yourself. There are also some things for which you are not responsible, which are primarily the concern of your client or group. Making a list of these areas may help you focus on your needs, and also highlight those areas which are essentially not your concern. Table 3 offers some suggestions.

Once you have made your list, it will be easier to focus on your own needs. There are some other issues that can be considered as well.

Educator responsibilities	Client responsibilities
Setting up the group — physically	Attending the group
Being available as a resource	Using the resources offered
Devising a program appropriate to client needs	Making use of the information provided
Taking account of differing learning styles in the group	Learning
Enabling clients to make decisions	Making the decisions
Being aware of own needs	Being aware of own physical needs
Being open, non-judgemental, flexible	Dealing with own emotional baggage
Getting the job done — providing what the group wants	Co-operating to get the best from what is on offer
Being resourceful	Being resourceful

TABLE 3: *Responsibilities of the educator and the client in the group learning situation.*

Learning how to separate our own lives from that of our clients is of primary importance. This means not becoming emotionally involved with their problems, not taking responsibility for their birth outcomes and finding ways of meeting our own needs without burdening our clients, or expecting them to support us. In a professional relationship, you must put your client's needs first, and find other avenues in which your needs can be met. Taking time out to realistically assess your own situation is a useful first step.

Most of us wear several 'hats'. We may be employed as midwives, physiotherapists, nurses or psychologists, for example, in addition to our work as childbirth educators. Many educators add parenting to that list, as well as wife and lover for our partners. Each of these areas involves special skills and perhaps training. Recognising the discrete nature of these tasks can be helpful in delineating responsibilities and keeping each compartment of our lives in perspective. If you are also a midwife, for example, this involves working in a maternity unit and assisting women to give birth. The competencies and politics involved in that job are not necessary for your role as an educator, which instead, entails teaching and group management. Similarly, your role as the mother of your children needs to be separated from your educator's work of presenting to adults in a group. Learning how to juggle these different hats and knowing which hat you are wearing at any given time is an important skill in itself, and one that is basic for a professional approach to childbirth education. One way of making it easier to change hats is to allow yourself a small break between each role — a few minutes to step out of your role as midwife or mother, put those attributes on a metaphorical shelf, before you take your childbirth educator's hat down in preparation for the approaching teaching session.

Debriefing your own birth and parenting experiences with a close friend or a professional counsellor could be important. When you are aware of your own feelings about these issues, and have had a chance to resolve any griefs you may be carrying, you will be in a better position to help others objectively. While it is appropriate for you to explore your experiences with a counsellor, it is not appropriate to discuss your births with women who are coming to you as a childbirth educator for information and support. If you need to discuss your own birth with someone (and what woman would not welcome such an opportunity?) find someone who can offer professional counselling, or a close friend unconnected with your work as an educator. Using an independent counsellor has another advantage — it will offer you valuable insights into the counselling role, and first-hand experience of the value of this approach to problem solving. Sorting out your own joys and sorrows about birth and parenting will not only help you personally, but will make unbiassed comment, non-judgemental responses and open-minded approaches to problem solving easier for you to model to the group. You will also find it easier to be clear about your teaching objectives and to evaluate the outcome of your work.

From time to time, you may find leading pre-natal groups quite stressful. Sometimes personal or family commitments intrude, creating pressures. At other times, your pre-natal group itself may be the source of stress, for example, being asked for information you don't have to hand, feeling rushed because of time constraints, having to deal with specific behaviours in the group (anxieties, fears, attention seeking behaviour etc.), needing to maintain rapport with people you don't like. It is impossible to predict when these stresses will occur and what effect they may have on you. If you have been stressed before, you may already know what this feels like and have developed ways of relieving the symptoms and reducing stress loads. If, however, you are finding that stress is a constant problem in your life, professional help may be necessary. Once you have identified the source(s) of your stress, you can devise strategies for reducing potential stressors in the future. Using the examples above: if you feel flustered because you are unsure of your information, you can read more widely, or seek answers from other health professionals; if you find time constraints frustrating, try setting group agendas to help prioritise and organise the time available; if you are nervous about certain topics because you find them uncomfortable, seek some help in resolving your own discomforts first, so you can approach these issues more calmly. Once again, the techniques you discover to be useful for yourself may have application in your work as an educator.

Take some time at the end of each class or group to review the session and debrief the behaviours, content covered and the responses of everyone present. This will help you to focus on particular stressors, deal with your own reactions and prepare for the next group. Try asking yourself:

- How was the group tonight? What did I notice about their energy/ involvement/interest?
- How did I feel about this session?
- What were the reactions to the material we covered?
- Did anything catch me by surprise?
- Which group members showed they had a special interest/need/concern/anxiety?
- How did I detect these needs?
- Were there topics that were omitted? Included?
- Would other teaching equipment/activities have helped my presentation?
- Were there any problems with the venue?
- What would I change if I could do it again?
- How will I make the next session different?
- What have I learned from this group?

If you were not very comfortable with your group, or felt dissatisfied with the outcome of the session (it didn't meet your own expectations), it may also be worthwhile taking a close look at your own motivations and needs regarding your teaching. There are many reasons why people take up the role of childbirth educator: to help women have 'better' births; to help women avoid certain birth outcomes; to have social contact with other parents; as a part-time job compatible with raising children; for stimulation and to 'keep the brain cells ticking over' before returning to full time work after raising young children; and so on. If, in addition, you have other personal needs, such as a need to have your group like you as a person, expecting that people will respond to your teaching in a certain way, being able to predict how women will respond in labour, having your group members form ongoing support systems after the session, etc. you will be working with quite a number of personal expectations that may be impossible to fulfil, and which therefore may become a source of potential stress.

Personal beliefs are also important to inspect from time to time as these can place further burdens on your ability to teach. An essential ingredient for effective teaching or counselling is a belief that people can solve their own problems. Similarly, if you want to empower others, then you need to believe that people can be empowered, that they have a right to be autonomous, and are able to take responsibility and show initiative. Without these basic beliefs, you may find yourself working at cross purposes — for example, trying to empower others, when in truth, you feel they are incapable of taking the necessary responsibility or action. As a result, you may feel stressed, and your group may feel confused, since it is likely that your non-verbal messages will conflict with your spoken communications. Sorting out your own position can lead to more effective teaching, an increase in group involvement, greater consistency in your message, and above all, can assist you to achieve your aims and objectives.

Another way to reduce stress is to develop your own support systems. A special friend, relative, partner or close colleague can be invaluable when you need someone to lean on. You need to debrief, vent feelings, be nurtured and loved too. Having your own needs met makes it easier to work with others. It is very difficult to avoid burn out if you have no mechanism for replenishing your own reserves of 'support' and 'caring'.

Many childbirth educators try to juggle young families, other full or part-time work, the needs of a partner, and some personal space with their work as educators. In addition, phone consultations, birth support work, attendance at conferences and workshops, constant background reading and basic class administration all add to the load. The resourcefulness and resilience of educators, faced with this kind of workload, is truly awesome, but it takes some organisation! It can also be a source of inspiration and example and of course, provides a good role model for the parents with whom you are working.

A sensible approach to proving the necessary back-up systems is vital if you are to be happy in your work, effective in your professional life, and relatively stress free. It is not a luxury to have help when working full time — most men in full time work, after all, have a wife to provide for them, and a woman with a full-time job (or two if you count raising a family and caring for a partner as full-time work) also needs support and practical assistance. You will need to assess you own resources and make appropriate arrangements according to your needs. Help with housework and child minding are likely to be top of the list, but do include personal needs, such as time out for recreation and pursuit of other interests. You may be able to pay for some of this additional help, or you may have to negotiate some sharing of household tasks with your partner. Learning to ask for help, negotiating with others for assistance, and finding ways of having your needs met are all useful skills for an educator to be able to model.

As you settle into your role of childbirth educator and develop the necessary skills, many of the stresses associated with teaching in the beginning will subside or be resolved. Background information and class content become familiar, you learn how to manage various group situations and counselling, presentation and teaching skills become more comfortable. You will still need to be ready for the unexpected! Your personal needs will also change as you grow and develop through your teaching. Allowing some time for personal reflection and acknowledging your own needs will help you keep your various roles in perspective.

Having now considered personal needs and resources, you will be better equipped to assist your clients with their needs. These may be many and varied.

Make no assumptions

Although each person in your group brings a whole raft of needs, wants and values to the group, don't make any assumptions about what these may be, especially in advance! Sometimes we hear statements such as 'She's the kind of person who always wants pain relief in labour', 'He won't make a very good support person for her — she should invite a friend if she wants practical help', 'People living in this area are so passive — they never ask questions in class', 'We never talk about . . . in my class because no-one ever wants to hear about it'. These are sure indications that assumptions are being made. How many times have mothers recounted being told in labour 'You are nowhere near being ready to push yet' and then given birth within minutes? These kinds of assumptions can prove very embarrassing, and threaten professional credibility!

Whenever we make assumptions especially about other people's feelings, beliefs, or predictable behaviours we risk disempowering others. By assuming we know what is happening inside another person or by predicting how they will behave, we are placing ourselves in a superior position, as if we have some special insight, cleverness or ability to accurately predict the future. We also run the risk of creating self-fulfilling prophesies in order to prove our hypothesis. There are lots of examples of this kind of thinking being put into action. In one famous experiment, a teacher was told that certain of her pupils were clever and others were not. She paid much more attention to the 'bright' children who rewarded her by improving their marks, even though they were no smarter than their peers. A woman who has been told through her pregnancy that she doesn't have to bear the pain of labour (as though she is incapable of managing her labour effectively) is much more vulnerable to accepting an epidural as soon as the labour begins, thereby fulfilling the predictor's prophesy that 'she was a wimp'.

To be truly supportive and empowering of other people, we must accept them as they are, feelings, behaviours and all. Stay open to their uniqueness and you will be better placed to offer alternatives and help them explore choices. If you have a fixed idea of what they are thinking or how they will react you will unconsciously promote behaviours that encourage the actions or thoughts you are expecting. It may give you pleasure to be 'right', but beware of the pitfalls — people are notoriously unpredictable and you will frequently be proven wrong in your guessing. It can be quite stressful to find you are constantly making mistakes!

Another problem with making assumptions is that in doing this we shut out the real needs of the other person, and miss an opportunity to learn from them. This is particularly important with pregnancy and birth, which are highly individual events, interpreted differently by each mother. If we assume how a woman will behave, or what she will want to know, or how her labour will unfold, or a whole host of other possibilities, then we risk losing the chance to learn from the wonderful variety of women's experiences.

Each time we work with a pregnant woman, the only assumption we can safely make is that she is an individual, with needs, reactions, feelings and responses that are uniquely hers. Our challenge is to help her discover her own individuality, and to make use of it during her pregnancy, birth and child rearing years.

When we abandon our assumptions, we are more open to other people. We can become curious, questioning, non-judgemental, all great assets in a group leader. When we are relaxed and open, our group will reflect this and the work of the group can proceed on an equitable and productive level.

CREATE A PERMISSIVE ATMOSPHERE

People are more willing to explore their own strengths and weaknesses and deal with their fears and anxieties if they sense trust and support and an environment of acceptance. It is easier to talk about deep feelings in a safe, non-judgemental atmosphere, when there is no fear of recrimination or adverse reaction from others who are present.

Developing these attributes is important for pre-natal groups, which may be the only opportunity members have to share feelings about pregnancy and birth with others in the same situation. It is likely that you will spend more time with them than any other health professional, thus you become their major resource as they develop parenting skills. In our culture, parenting is often an isolating experience, so the development of mutually supportive social networks with other parents can be a practical outcome of pre-natal classes. These social networks are more likely to develop if there has been honesty, openness and trust in the pre-natal group.

The onus of establishing a permissive atmosphere in your group will initially rest with you. As the group begins to interact socially, it can develop its own framework where members feel trust and mutual respect. The first steps, however, must come from you, as the leader.

The first impression you create will have a major impact. You need to be warm, friendly, relaxed and hospitable. The first time you meet together, try acting as though you are hosting a social gathering of people whom you don't know. Introduce people around, make some small talk, establish a relaxed and social setting from the start. If you set your room up as a classroom, stand at the front, talk at people rather than with them, you will instantly create a feeling of formality and distance. Offering refreshments right at the start can make it easier to socialise, as people often feel more relaxed with something to eat and drink in their hands while they circulate and meet others.

An activity that can help set the tone and working environment for the group is to set 'group rules' in the first session. This activity is described in Part 3. Having a set of guidelines for acceptable behaviours among group members establishes a framework for the interactions that will follow. Ground rules enable members to work together more productively, and can help defuse potentially difficult situations. Of course, you too must obey the ground rules. If you override the guidelines agreed by your group you risk setting yourself up for conflict and possibly alienating individuals. It may appear to your group that there are two sets of rules, one for them and another for you. For example, if the group has decided that everyone's opinion is to be respected, you have to avoid making comments that could be construed as judgemental, especially in the early life of the group, when people are forming working relationships with each other.

As the session develops, maintain a very welcoming manner. Be aware of your facial expressions, your thoughts and reactions during discussions. Sometimes, our accidental non-verbal responses create a distance or strain in the group, particularly when people feel strange and don't know each other. In the first session, everyone is especially sensitive, and learning how to keep a 'poker face' is an important attribute of a good leader or counsellor.

The language we use also conveys our feelings on many issues, so be aware of what you are saying and notice the impact of your words on the listener.

When members of the group do start talking about their worries or concerns, or raise private issues for discussion, either in private or in the group, it is imperative that you maintain their confidentiality. This is particularly important to the group process and to the level of trust that exists in the group. For example, it is quite likely that from time to time you may have a doctor, midwife, other health professional, or a well known public figure in your group. You may know of this person's identity in advance, perhaps through the booking procedure for the class. When everyone is introducing themselves in the first class, take special note of how much each person reveals to the group. If they announce their job or title, then you have permission to mention it later if it is appropriate, but if nothing is said about their background, then you must maintain the confidentiality of this information or you will lose their trust. Never use people with relevant qualifications to verify or expand on your information, without their permission. Constant deference to their expertise will also undermine your position as group leader.

Similarly, group members may reveal something to you in private, or you may be aware that they have special needs (such as a particular medical condition or a social circumstance) from information you have received from other sources. Don't reveal this kind of information to others, or the group, without the expressed permission from the person concerned.

When you are talking about 'delicate', potentially frightening or embarrassing topics, ease gently into the subject and check with the group that it is acceptable to discuss the issue. Having their permission to proceed will show that you respect their right to shape the agenda, and to deal with potentially difficult subjects when they are ready. It is much easier to talk about uncomfortable topics, such as unexpected outcomes, if the group can nominate when it is to be discussed, and if everyone's feelings are acknowledged and respected.

TRY COUNSELLING, NOT TEACHING TECHNIQUES

The key to making all this happen is to use counselling skills rather than teaching techniques as a group leader. As you develop your skills as a childbirth educator, you will find that you are spending less time talking and much more time listening to the people in your group. This is an important step in the empowerment process, since listening is an essential tool for discovering what parents would like to achieve with pregnancy, birth and parenthood. When you have identified these goals you are in a better position to assist them solve problems, decide on plans of action, and make the inevitable decisions that having choice dictates. None of this will happen if you just tell people what to do or give advice.

It takes time to develop counselling skills and they can only be acquired through practice. Joining groups yourself or seeking counselling experiences for your own needs are useful ways to learn. Counselling is a broad term for a collection of smaller, micro skills that collectively form a particular style of interaction with others. Many of the basic micro skills can be used in pre-natal classes to make your leadership more effective.

LISTENING

You don't need to talk all the time! There will certainly be times when information needs to be given in short lecture formats, but try and keep these to a minimum, perhaps for topics likely to be unfamiliar such as drugs in labour, obstetric procedures etc. Much of the time, your group members will already know something about the topic under discussion, and you can draw this out by using 'open' questions. These begin with words such as:

HOW

- 'How did you find out about . . .?'
- 'How did it happen that . . .?'

WHEN

- 'When did you feel . . .?'
- 'When . . . happened, how did . . .?'

WHERE

- 'Where would you expect . . .?'
- 'Where were you when . . .?'

WHAT

- 'In what way would you . . .?'
- 'What makes you think that . . .?'

'Closed' questions invite a simple 'yes/no' response and do nothing to further the discussion, which stops dead. They are often designed to enlist support for the questioner's point of view, or to gain agreement for a particular plan of action. Using these openings for your questions disempowers people. They often start with:

- 'Did . . .'

- 'Isn't it true that . . .'
- 'Don't you feel/agree/like . . .'
- 'Isn't it wonderful/sad/exciting . . .'
- 'Would/wouldn't . . .'

Starting a question with the word 'why' can force people into taking a defensive position, to justify their actions or thoughts. A 'why' question often results in an answer that begins with 'because'. This tends to close off the conversation and create a distance between the parties.

When people respond to a question you have asked, listen carefully to what is being said, not just for assessing the accuracy of the answer, but to pick up the feelings being expressed.

CLARIFYING

The next step is to check that you have heard correctly. Don't make assumptions! Checking can be done by reflecting the answer back to the speaker in slightly different words (paraphrasing) which will let the speaker know that you have been listening carefully. This indicates your interest and support, and offers the chance to correct any misinterpretations you may have made. You can address the feelings as well as the facts in this way. Clarifying can be achieved by saying:

- 'It sounds as though you were upset/excited/surprised by . . .'
- 'I get the feeling you thought that . . .'
- 'Am I right in thinking that you . . .'
- 'So you felt that . . .'

With this approach, the conversation will often move forward with further information or feelings being revealed and the issue being discussed in greater depth. Sometimes it will become apparent that there is a problem underlying the issue that would be best resolved. As a counsellor, you may be able to clarify the problem and assist in moving your client towards resolving the situation. You could try saying, for example:

- 'It seems, from what you are saying that there may be a problem here . . .'
- 'Would it help if you were able to . . . ?'
- 'Why do you think . . . is happening?'

Once a problem has been identified, you can then help your client explore various solutions, as described later in Part 3. While you are doing this, avoid giving advice, and use reflective listening and clarification techniques to keep the issue firmly centred on your client. As soon as you offer advice, the focus will shift to you, and your client becomes less important.

If you are asked for your advice, think very carefully before jumping in with lots of suggestions or strongly worded comment ('If I were you I would . . .', 'I would recommend . . .', 'If you want my advice, I can only say that the best way to go would be to . . .'). Often, when someone is seeking your advice, it doesn't necessarily mean that they have no ideas of their own, or even a strong preference for a particular plan of action. It may just mean that they are having a struggle with the process of making a decision, and would appreciate some guidance. Check it out! Don't assume they know absolutely nothing, and want to be told what to do, especially by an 'expert'. Try a comment such as:

- 'Yes, it is hard to decide when there are several ways of approaching this problem. What have you been considering?'
- 'I guess it is hard to make a decision sometimes'
- 'I can see you are having some trouble making up your mind. What would make it easier for you to decide?'

Listening, clarifying, and problem solving are all basic to the counselling process and help to keep your focus on your client and their needs. This, in turn, is central to the empowerment process.

This kind of approach works very well with individuals but can also work with groups. By using opportunities for the group to work on common concerns it encourages the group to take responsibility for working together and increases members' confidence that they can come up with their own ideas — useful preparation for what will happen in the hospital, when they are on their own, and needing to be independent. For example, instead of presenting the group with a list of self-help ideas for labour, you could ask them to work in small groups to compile suggestions for relaxation aids and a list of practical items they could take to hospital to make labour more comfortable. As they share their lists with the larger group, your task is to listen to the suggestions carefully and clarify obscure points or impractical suggestions (e.g. 'How do you think the candles might be viewed by the hospital staff?', 'How were you going to use the . . .?', 'What do you think might happen if you tried to . . . in the labour ward?'). This is a better approach than 'approving' or 'disapproving' of their ideas based on your own view or mental list of approved labour aids. By supporting their ideas you have left them in an empowered position, and you have avoided taking over as an expert. Your group's creative list might also give you some food for thought!

Empower your clients to make decisions

Raising children involves making lots of decisions. It is a fact of life that every day, parents face choices, problems to be solved and situations that need resolving if the family is to function at even a basic level. Everyone has to be fed, clothed and housed, and the relationships in a family need to be acknowledged and accommodated. The need to make decisions is one of the responsibilities involved in childrearing, and is one of the major stressors faced by new parents.

People who are used to taking responsibility in other areas of their lives, who are familiar with the processes of making decisions and who have experienced taking charge of a situation in order to effect an outcome, are often better equipped to adapt to this aspect of parenting. Those who have relied on others to make decisions for them may find it difficult to cope with the pressures of parenthood. For them, the constant necessity to make decisions about child rearing issues and the resultant burden of responsibility can be very difficult to manage.

It could be argued that the single most important skill needed by a new parent is the ability to make decisions. Every newly pregnant woman is immediately faced with dilemmas and choices that will affect her health and that of her baby. Every new parent discovers that they are 'on their own' after the birth since in our culture parents are expected to be self-reliant. It makes sense that we offer expectant parents the chance to develop skills in making decisions from the beginning of the pregnancy, to allow as much time as possible for them to practise before they find themselves being 'left holding the baby'.

Fortunately there are many opportunities for parents to develop and practise these skills because there will be a number of situations that arise during the pregnancy and birth where choices can be made. Indeed, since people become parents the moment a baby is conceived, it is appropriate that they begin making decisions right away, as there are many issues such as lifestyle changes and selecting maternity care that need to be considered for their impact on the future health of themselves and their baby.

The single most important decision that prospective parents will make, in terms of the outcome of the birth and the potential future health of their child, concerns the choice of caregiver for the pregnancy, labour and birth. Research has clearly shown that the attitudes, philosophy and practices of the main caregiver present during labour and birth will shape the management of the event and have a huge impact on the quality of the experience for each parent, and also for the baby. Research has shown, for example, that a midwife, with

An informed choice is one in which
Accurate information is provided — the information presented is based on 'state of the art' knowledge.
The specific points where choice is available are detailed and outlined.
The advantages and disadvantages of the various options are given.
Enough time is given for consideration of the physical and psychological implications of each choice.
There is information included about any potential risks, flowing from specific decisions, presented in a sensitive, non-threatening manner.
Crisis decisions — based on information which is unavailable to the parent(s) — are delegated to the medical attendants.
Emotional support is available, regardless of the decision made.
Evaluation is made to ensure that information is understood.

TABLE 4: *The concept of an informed choice.*

a training and philosophy centred on birth as a normal bodily process, approaches assisting a woman in labour differently from a doctor, who tends to view birth from his training in the medical model of treating illness. A midwife is more likely to assume that the labour is going well unless it is demonstrably not the case, whereas a doctor is more likely to assume there will be a problem, and demand proactive intervention, just in case problems occur later. Therefore, the decision a woman makes about who will assist her at the time of the birth could be of fundamental importance to the future emotional and physical health of herself and her baby.

A woman, pregnant for the first time, has many needs: for practical support; for positive input and encouragement; to have her confidence in being a mother reinforced; to nurture intuitive feelings; to build self esteem; and to acquire parenting skills. A woman needs to be involved in her own care, enabled to make decisions, supported in her choices at all times, and to be made to feel important and competent. Caregivers need to be chosen with these needs in mind, and parents may need help to choose wisely.

Of course, it would be much easier to assist parents to make this decision if they sought help early enough in the pregnancy. By the time expectant parents arrive in your pre-natal classes, these decisions have usually been made some time ago, and a relationship has been forged between the woman and her caregiver. She may not be entirely happy with this relationship and even have doubts about the care being given, but she often feels that a decision has been made and that it is irrevocable. Even if she does want to investigate alternatives, she may not know how to do this, and may feel nervous about potential conflict or embarrassed by perceived social difficulties. Helping parents make the vital decision about choice of caregiver is one of the most powerful arguments in favour of early pregnancy classes. Providing information about how to seek second opinions and change doctors is essential later in the pregnancy, if we are to be supportive of consumerism and choice in childbirth.

There will be further issues faced by parents that offer opportunities for exercising a right of choice, firstly during the pregnancy. Some of these are:

- Choice of caregiver — midwife, GP or obstetrician?
- The place of birth — home, hospital or birth centre?
- Lifestyle decisions — nutrition, smoking, alcohol.
- Pre-natal diagnostic tests — ultrasound, tests for fetal well-being, termination of pregnancy.
- Treatments for specific maternal health problems — e.g. diabetes, high blood pressure, vaginal infections, herpes.
- Treatment for fetal health problems — e.g. intrauterine growth retardation, threatened premature birth.
- Induction for non-medical reasons.
- Alternative managements for breech or twins births . . .

DURING THE LABOUR, NEW DILEMMAS ARISE

- Initiation of labour — spontaneous or induced?
- Augmentation or natural progression?
- Management following rupture of membranes, with no contractions?
- Drugs or self help remedies for pain relief?
- Electronic fetal monitoring or auscultation by the midwife?
- Position for second stage?
- Management of third stage . . .

AND IMMEDIATELY AFTER THE BIRTH

- Vitamin K administration.
- Circumcision.
- Early discharge or longer stay in hospital?
- Breast or bottle feeding . . .

MAKING A DECISION

There are a number of steps in the process of making a decision.

DEFINING THE PROBLEM

Being clear about the nature of the problem is essential. It is difficult to weigh up various solutions when you are not quite sure what the basic problem is, or even if it is a problem at all. It is also helpful to identify if the problem is one that could be described as 'yours' or whether the solution or resolution of the situation really lies with someone else. One way to clarify the nature of the problem is to ask some basic questions:

- 'What seems to be the trouble here?'
- 'Is this an important issue for me — does it really matter?'
- 'Will the quality of my life be irrevocably damaged if I don't sort this out?'
- 'Is this a problem that only I can deal with or is it basically up to someone else? Whose problem is this anyway?'

Once you have decided that there is a problem that must or should be resolved, then the next step is to determine a desired outcome.

WHAT DO I WANT INSTEAD?

Having a clear goal makes it easier to formulate a reasonable plan of action to achieve the outcome you want. Note that outcomes are often unpredictable, since they may ultimately be affected by forces or conditions over which you have no control. For example, a new mother may have a major problem in managing to juggle the needs of her baby and get a meal on the table when she and her partner need it. She may decide that this is a problem only she can solve, since her partner is at work all day and they can't afford take-away food very often, so she decides that she will begin preparing the meal earlier in the day to avoid a last minute rush. This may be a very workable solution, but she can't predict if the chicken will take longer to defrost than she planned, or if there will be a major storm and a subsequent blackout!

Once you have an idea of the outcome you want, it is easier to envisage possible pathways towards the goal. Try and be clear about the outcome — is it a behavioural change that you wish to see, or is it a specific thing you want to achieve?

HOW CAN I ACHIEVE THE GOAL?

Exploring the various avenues available that may help you achieve your goal is the next step. It is useful to try and think up several possibilities — that way you know you have canvassed various options, and you will have a fall-back position available if the chosen option does not achieve your outcome. As you consider the various options available, you need to check several points for each one:

- 'Is this realistic? Is it within my power to make this option work?'

  For example, annoying behaviour in a partner may be so entrenched that it is unrealistic to expect them to change. In addition, it is not within your power to make them change, since they would have to do the work, not you.

- 'If I choose this option, might it cause further problems, perhaps for others?'

  Choosing a course of action that would harm another person is not justifiable behaviour. Sometimes others can be hurt unexpectedly (an unpredictable outcome), but making a choice that you know will have a likely effect on others does not demonstrate a responsible approach. Many mothers choose to use drugs in labour because they don't know that this short term pain relief in labour will have an effect on their unborn baby. Most mothers, knowing of these potential side effects, will consider other less invasive pain relief options, to protect their baby from harm. Sometimes women will have to weigh up their comfort against the health of their baby — a difficult decision.

'WHAT ARE MY PRIORITIES?'

Ranking options according to priorities can be useful. There may be options that will give a short term solution but not address the problem in the longer term. There may be options that could be tried out more easily or speedily than others. Listing the options in terms of their ease of implementation could be helpful at this stage.

'LET'S TAKE THE PLUNGE!'

This is decision time. Of all the possible choices to be made, one has to be selected. It may not turn out to be the best one, but at least you know there are others than can be used if needed.

'Did it work?'

Have you achieved the outcome you wanted? If you did, then you no longer have the problem. If your first choice has left you not much further ahead, or even created a new problem, then you will have to go back and choose another of your options. Trial and error is often the way we learn best, and experience is always valuable.

As you can see, there are a number of steps in making a decision. Most people will go through this kind of checklist very quickly, particularly with practice. Understanding the steps involved is important, as it gives insight into the way to tackle problem solving, and when a really big problem arrives, consciously using this process can be helpful. It may not be too hard to quickly decide what clothes to wear in the morning, but making a decision about which hospital to choose for the birth of your baby may take careful thought.

Describing the problem solving mechanism and allowing plenty of opportunities for practice in class may be the most important aspect of your teaching. Assisting your clients to establish goals for themselves and having them work out ways they can be achieved is a basic tool of empowerment. In our health system, decisions are usually made by others, often calling themselves 'experts', and as a result many parents are disempowered and rendered helpless. A decision, even an unpleasant one, taken by the person involved rather than imposed by others, will leave the person empowered. In the face of a crisis, a mother may request a caesarean, which she had wanted to avoid earlier, because she now knows her baby needs rescuing quickly. A caesarean that is imposed by a caregiver, without a demonstrable need, may leave the woman feeling cheated and angry.

Many people have difficulties making decisions. Taking control in one's own life is a novel concept for some. Perhaps their opportunities for making personal choices have been limited, and they have little experience of making major decisions. Some people deliberately avoid situations where they will have to choose, as their self-esteem is so low that they fear failure. Others seek protection, choosing to avoid making any decisions, in a child-like approach to life. Type of personality, previous life experience, opportunity, life situation and current circumstances all have an impact on the way adults approach the solving of problems they encounter.

For some people, the fact that they have made a decision is the most important aspect of the exercise. A person who constantly allows others to decide, acts on other people's advice and relies on being led by 'experts' may find it very threatening to be asked to decide for themselves. This may be exacerbated in situations where the person has little or no previous experience or information on which they can draw.

Many women, pregnant for the first time, are confronted by a bewildering array of new experiences, at a time when they may be feeling emotionally vulnerable and have little access to information that can be readily understood. It is no wonder that many feel at a disadvantage. It is easy for others to take over and dictate courses of action. If this happens women may feel disempowered and their self esteem may suffer. It is sometimes hard for health professionals to recognise the effects of their 'rescue' actions on individuals in these circumstances, and sometimes even harder for them to break familiar patterns of behaviour in order to benefit their clients. Making decisions for others, and solving problems for other people is the basic premise of the medical model of health care, which is totally inappropriate in maternity care. As an educator, you are in a position to have an impact on this situation, through deliberate inclusion of problem solving exercises in your classes, and unequivocal support of your clients and their decisions. Being able to make a decision and take responsibility flows from feeling empowered, and enabling pregnant women and their partners to feel comfortable with these actions may be the most effective aspect of your teaching.

EVERYONE MAKES MISTAKES

Making a decision does not imply that the correct or best decision will always be made. Everyone can look back at decisions made in the past and wish they had chosen better options. It is easy to be wise with the benefit of hindsight. This needs to be understood and discussed as part of the problem solving mechanism. Many decisions can be reversed, or corrective action can be taken later to improve an unexpected outcome. Sometimes events may turn out badly as a result of a decision and having to live with the consequences may be an inevitable result. In this situation, however, it is rare that there are no positive gains from the experience, even if it is only the fact that a deliberate move was made to affect the outcome (a decision was made) rather than just allowing events to unfold or permitting someone else to take control.

Learning from one's mistakes is an important part of growing up and exercising responsibility. Being able to admit one's mistakes is harder, and a healthy sign of maturity. It is easier for both of these to occur in a supportive environment. As a parent, accepting the mistakes of one's children and encouraging experimentation in a supportive environment in which a child can assume responsibility helps them develop into capable, responsible adults. Many people have not had this kind of upbringing, and so, faced with the need to make a decision, feel insecure, dependent, and anxious about making a mistake.

Your attitude as an educator, particularly in relation to supporting the decisions made by your clients, is very important. Having explained choices available, answered their questions, ensured that they understand the information and stood by them as they made their decisions, you must be prepared to accept that sometimes people will choose to do things in a different way from you. It can be hard to avoid the 'told you so' syndrome, either consciously or unconsciously (remember your non-verbal behaviour here!) and you will need to debrief yourself when you have helped your clients to debrief their experiences. Having clear goals for classes will help you avoid the trap of inadvertently pushing people to emulate your own achievements in birth. When you have a client centred approach to your teaching, it is much easier to accept that mistakes will be made, people will do things differently from you, and that the important gains are in areas such as the ability to make decisions rather than the decisions themselves.

FURTHER READING

Baldwin R. & Palmarini T. 1986, *Pregnant Feelings*, Celestial Arts, California, USA.

Hunter D., Bailey A., & Taylor B. 1992, *The Zen of Groups*, Tandem Press, New Zealand.

Geldard D. 1993, *Basic Personal Counselling*, Prentice Hall.

Raphael-Leff J. 1990, *Psychological Process of Childbearing*, Chapman & Hall, UK.

PART TWO

EXPLORING ANATOMY AND PHYSIOLOGY

CHAPTER 4

DESIGN FOR BIRTH

DEVELOPING YOUR UNDERSTANDING

Childbirth educators need to have a thorough knowledge of the anatomy and physiology of pregnancy, labour and birth before they begin teaching pre-natal classes. Pregnant women are curious about what is happening inside their bodies, and will ask many questions. This is an important part of feeling empowered, as with background knowledge a woman is better equipped to ask questions, discuss alternatives and make decisions.

This manual focuses on those aspects of physiology and anatomy that relate to normal labour and birth. There are many variations on this theme, and a wide variety of behaviours and conditions that could be included in a general description of 'normal'. In addition to the information described here, educa-tors will need to be familiar with potential complications in pregnancy and birth, and be aware of the choices and options available to women in those cir-cumstances. Similarly, a wide knowledge of obstetric procedures and pain relieving drugs is essential, and it is important to keep this knowledge up to date and based on current research findings. This can be achieved through subscription to professional journals or a comprehensive reader's service such as MIDIRS Midwifery Digest, accessing a computer database such as the Cochrane Collaboration Pregnancy and Childbirth Updates on Disk or using comprehensive references such as *Effective Care in Pregnancy and Childbirth* by Murray Enkin, Marc Kierse and Ian Chalmers, or the summary volume *A Guide to Effective Care in Pregnancy and Childbirth*, by the same authors. Useful references are listed at the end of this chapter.

All women are born with the ability to give birth. Very early in fetal life, innate instinct and knowledge on how to survive and reproduce is embedded in the primitive part of the brain known as the hypothalamus. All animals have these essential behaviours which are designed to ensure perpetuation of the species. These behaviours involve automatic responses, triggered by stimuli that may be consciously recognised or aroused by unconscious awareness. Survival behaviours can be observed in newborns, as they instinctively find the nipple, engage the mother's attention and stimulate her nurturing responses. Reproductive behaviours appear at puberty as maturity develops and the body is prepared for the ability to recreate life. A woman, having conceived, has little control over the forces that govern and regulate her pregnancy and the development of her baby — the whole system is designed to operate automatically, to increase the likelihood of survival of the baby regardless of the mother's actions. Similarly, the birth process, under the influence of instinct and the drive for reproductive success, is largely shaped by automatic responses to unconscious hormonal interactions.

Therefore, we have no need to teach women *how* to give birth as they already have this information available. It is helpful to understand the process, however, as a means of encouraging insights into personal needs during labour, and the factors which influence these automatic responses.

For childbirth educators, a thorough working knowledge of the anatomy and physiology of birth is vital. It is impossible to teach convincingly if you are not familiar or comfortable with the subject material. Having a theoretical knowledge of the birth process is insufficient to inspire and motivate others — it takes experience of the nuances of behaviour, the ability to explain patterns of responses, and an understanding of the 'big picture' of hormonal and physical interplay within which to interpret the string of smaller reactions produced by labouring women. These insights come from observations of births and a questioning mind — 'Why did she react in that way?', 'What is really happening here?'. A thorough theoretical knowledge provides a foundation from which you can explore and interpret your observations.

Being with women who are labouring normally (no drips, monitors, drugs or restrictions on movement or behaviours) is the best way to learn about birth. Once you have an appreciation of the enormous variety of women's reactions to labour, you will be better equipped to empower others. Without this basis for your work, you risk appearing insincere, and unconvinced about womens' innate birthing abilities. If the foundations for your work in childbirth education appear shaky then you will have difficulty enabling your clients to construct a solid framework from which they can discover their own needs.

This section of the book is designed, therefore, to expand your knowledge of the theory of normal physiological birth. It is not intended to be comprehensive, but to address those areas of special interest is relation to active birth. There is much to be discovered about hormonal interplays and personal response during labour. Use this information as a starting point for your own observations of labour and birth. In addition, read widely, talk to women who have given birth and sharpen your powers of observation. These are valuable, and necessary, adjuncts to learning more about the special creative powers possessed by women.

THE ROLE OF THE PELVIS IN LABOUR

The pelvis is, quite literally, the seat of all the action in labour. The bony cradle that supports the internal organs and the growing baby during pregnancy also forms an encircling ring, a tunnel, through which the baby passes to be born. Male and female pelves are slightly different in shape, reflecting the need for the female pelvis to accommodate a baby as it is being born.

There are aspects of pelvic construction that are cleverly designed to enhance the passage of the baby:

- the shape and position of the main joints (the sacroiliac and pubic joints) enable the bones to move in ways that increase the internal diameters of the pelvis and therefore, its capacity,
- the curved shape of the sacrum serves to direct the baby towards the exit,
- the inferior pubic rami are flared forwards to assist the passage of the baby under the pubic arch,
- the joints are held in place by a system of ligaments that allow movement between the bones of the pelvic girdle. These ligaments (and all the other ligaments supporting joints in the body) are sensitive to the hormone relaxin, produced during pregnancy, which increases their elasticity and thus movement at the joints. When combined with body weight and an upright posture, the added flexibility of the joints can increase internal capacity of the pelvic outlet by up to 28%.

Inspection of a model pelvis will reveal these important design features. Working with these attributes to make the most of pelvic capacity is explained in the exercise 'Learning about the pelvis' in Part 3 of this book.

Women have traditionally made use of these special qualities of the pelvis in labour. Illustrations from old midwifery and obstetric textbooks show women adopting a variety of positions for birth that take advantage of pelvic design. Indeed, if they had not made use of their bodies' innate capacity for birth, in many cases their babies would not have been born. Some texts show women in extraordinary positions for birth, which appear at first glance to be more akin to torture than reproductive behaviours. If inspected closely however, it becomes apparent that these positions were often adopted in situations of extreme difficulty, where the mother and/or the baby were at risk. Without access to an operating theatre for a life-saving caesarean section, midwives were forced to become inventive, and, without necessarily understanding the physical theory behind their actions, drew on experience and enlarged the passage with exaggerated postures that increased the chances of the baby being born alive.

Many women are concerned that their pelvic capacity may be limited and that they will therefore have difficulty in giving birth, perhaps even requiring a caesarean section. Women who have had a caesarean birth are especially at risk in this respect, as many have been given 'cephalo pelvic disproportion' or 'dystocia' as a reason for the caesarean section. Since the pelvis is an elasticised system of bones, especially during pregnancy, static pictures obtained through ultrasound or x-rays will not show the true capacity of the pelvis during labour. Therefore, pelvimetry measurements must be treated with caution. Even manual examinations made by the midwife or doctor will not reveal the true picture — only the forces created by the mother and baby during birth will allow the pelvis to open to its full potential. This may take some time, but is the only true way of exploring the 'fit' between the mother and baby during birth.

The thigh bones (femurs) form levers against the sides of the pelvis, an action that is increased by opening the legs, leaning forwards and supporting the body weight on the legs. A pregnant woman has the additional weight of the baby which adds to the gravitational effect when she is upright. Her weight can be taken on either the feet, knees or thighs, for example, when sitting on a birth stool. To obtain maximum benefit in labour, the pelvic bones must not be restricted (for example, by sitting on the bones), and the woman should be able to move freely to adjust the drive angle of the baby inside the pelvis, and to increase her pelvic capacity through her body movements. The need to brace her upper body and/or to have solid ground against which to bear weight may be symptomatic of instinctive behaviour designed to help her make space for the emerging baby. Perhaps this is one reason why women, labouring in the bath, sometimes feel the need to get out as they enter the second stage of labour: they may need the full effect of their body's weight and gravity to create room for the baby.

POSTURE AND GRAVITY

Once labour has begun, the pressure of the presenting part of the baby on the dilating cervix helps to trigger the release of oxytocin in the body and maintain the labour contractions. The presenting part will be better applied to the cervix if the mother is in a vertical position, so that the weight of the baby increases the effect of the gravity. Labour has been shown to be shorter if the mother is upright.

A labouring woman will also find that the contractions are much less painful if the weight of the baby and uterus is pressing downwards on the soft pelvic floor muscles. When she lies down, particularly on her back or her side, the weight of the heavy uterus and its contents presses on other muscles, tissues and organs in such a way that it is difficult for her to get comfortable. Many women will have already noticed this when they have tried to sleep in the last weeks of their pregnancy and found it very difficult to get comfortable in a recumbent position.

During second stage, the effect of gravity is even more important. Whilst the uterus is quite capable of expelling a baby solely through its own action, encouraging the mother into a suitable vertical position will speed up progress and enhance the uterine action. It is much more difficult for the uterus to expel the baby if the mother is lying on her back because the baby has to be forced horizontally and then vertically upwards, directly against gravity. Similarly, with lateral positions, the baby needs to be moved horizontally, and the effect of gravity is of no assistance in the process. When a mother is upright, gravity acts in the same direction as the driving force of the uterus, and a mother in such a position often finds that her need to push is reduced. Taking advantage of gravity can be very helpful for women who have had an epidural which has not quite worn off, and in whom the pushing reflex is reduced or absent. It is also beneficial for those mothers who are very tired after a long and arduous labour. If these women can be supported in a suitable upright position, then the uterus can do the necessary work and the mother's need to provide the primary force through pushing efforts is reduced.

Being upright offers additional advantages. It is easier for a woman to release pelvic floor muscles and perineal tissues when she is upright, as this is a familiar action. Every time she uses the toilet, she releases these muscles, and when moving her bowels she utilises a pushing urge. The difference between pushing in an upright position and pushing in a horizontal one can easily be demonstrated: imagine trying to open your bowels using a bedpan while lying down. Wouldn't it be easier if you were able to sit up or straddle a toilet? The key elements in this example are the links between familiarity and posture — you are used to moving your bowels in a vertical position and it requires no conscious thought. The muscle fibres of the pelvic floor are at their optimal length for relaxation, and this reduces stress on these tissues and the likelihood of excessive stretching or tearing. Taking advantage of these kinds of automatic responses in labour increases a woman's ability to act instinctively.

Being vertical enables a woman in labour to move freely and experiment with different positions. Many heavily pregnant women find it almost impossible to turn over once recumbent, a fact they have discovered during the last weeks of the pregnancy. When upright, however, it is easy to bend and turn, to shift the body's weight, and to move from one position to another. Women use these kinds of movements automatically in response to the pressures and forces of labour, provided they stay upright, not anchored to a bed. There are no 'right' or 'wrong' positions for labour, only those that a woman finds comfortable and efficient for her. Encouraging women to adopt certain positions or directing her movements in any way, whilst often well-intentioned, may detract from her sense of autonomy in labour. A woman's companions during labour have a role in creating a permissive atmosphere in which she is free to experiment, in ensuring no disturbances to her natural rhythm and in protecting her right to adopt any posture that she feels is helpful to progress.

Further reading

Balaskas J. 1989, *The New Active Birth*, Harper Collins.

Flynn A., Kelly J., Hollins G. & Lynch P. 1978, 'Ambulation in labour', *BMJ*, August 1978, pp. 591–593.

Gardosi J., Hutson W. & B-Lynch C. 1989, 'Randomised controlled trial of squatting in the second stage of labour', *Lancet*, July 8, pp. 74–77.

Gardosi J., Sylvester S. & B-Lynch C. 1989, 'Alternative positions in the second stage of labour: a randomised controlled trial', *Brit J of Obstet & Gyn*, vol. 96, pp. 1290–1296.

Grant J. 1987, 'Reassessing second stage', *Assoc of Chartered Physiotherapists in Obstets and Gynaec Journal*, no. 60, pp. 26–30.

Limberg A. & Smulders B. 1993, *Women Giving Birth*, Celestial Arts, California.

Paciornik M. 1990, 'Arguments against episiotomy and in favour of squatting for birth', *Birth*, vol. 17, no. 2.

Roberts J. 1989, 'Maternal position during first stage of labour', in *Effective Care in Pregnancy and Childbirth*, eds I. Chalmers, M. Enkin & M. Keirse, Oxford University Press, Oxford, pp. 883–892.

Roberts J., Mendez-Bauer C. & Wodell D. 1983, 'The effects of maternal position on uterine contractility and efficiency', *Birth*, vol. 10, no. 4.

Russell J. 1982, 'The rationale of primitive delivery positions', *BMJ*, vol. 89, pp. 712–715.

Sleep J., Roberts J. & Chalmers I. 1989, 'Care during the second stage of labour' in *Effective Care in Pregnancy and Childbirth*, eds I. Chalmers, M. Enkin & M. Keirse, Oxford University Press, Oxford.

CHAPTER 5

THE HORMONAL SYSTEM

It is the action of the hormones that governs the physiology of birth. From the moment of conception a woman's hormonal balance changes and the interplay of the special pregnancy hormones, together with those that regulate other metabolic functions, affect her whole physical functioning and well being.

Many women regard their 'hormones' as a problem, a notion that is often reinforced by the dismissive excuses made for their behaviour as being 'hormonal', as though this was some kind of curse rather than an integral part of reproduction. In fact, a healthy balance of hormones is necessary for the maintenance of the pregnancy, and a smooth flow of chemical messages between mother and baby regulates fetal development, the initiation of labour and its safe conclusion in birth.

Helping women to understand how the basic hormones work and their importance in a successful pregnancy and birth is an important element of a childbirth educator's work.

There are many players on the hormonal stage, and we will focus here only on those with leading roles in labour. In choosing to explore oxytocin, endorphin and catecholamines (adrenalin) we can canvass the reasons for the behaviours displayed by labouring women and identify major influences on successful outcomes. When discussing practical management strategies, it is to these hormones and the factors that influence their production that we can look for inspiration and guidance in developing the most appropriate labouring climate for a woman. These three hormones are central and essential elements of normal, physiological birth.

OXYTOCIN

Oxytocin has often been called 'the hormone of love', as it is the main hormone in every reproductive response in both men and women, and fulfils a number of interconnected functions. It is produced in the hypothalamic region of the brain and is stored and secreted by the posterior pituitary gland.

Ferguson first described, in 1941, the reflex whereby oxytocin is released from the posterior pituitary gland in response to stimulation of certain sites, integral to reproductive behaviours. Although his name has been largely forgotten in this context, practitioners will be familiar with the clinical application of his work, and its vital importance in the reproductive processes.

It causes uterine contractions throughout the reproductive life of women, especially during menstruation, pregnancy, labour and birth. The milk ejection reflex is initiated by oxytocin, released in response to the baby's suckling. Less well-known effects of oxytocin include:

- Its presence triggers caretaking behaviours: males become more protective of females and in return females provide comfort and support for males. This closeness may be an important mechanism for ensuring that offspring have two parents as caretakers.
- During sexual intercourse, oxytocin increases the motility of the fallopian tubes, which influences sperm transport.
- Sperm transport is also assisted by the in-sucking action of the uterus caused by oxytocin driven contractions of the uterus.
- The presence of oxytocin can enhance the manufacture of sperm and encourage early ovulation in females.
- Skin temperature is affected by the presence of oxytocin — the body and particularly the breast becomes warmer.
- Following orgasm, and the release of oxytocin, anxiety states and depression are reduced. Orgasm makes you feel good!
- The surge of oxytocin during orgasm or masturbation can cause a lactating female to release her milk.
- Oxytocin release during lactation has been shown to induce maternal, nurturing behaviours.
- During breastfeeding, the spurts of oxytocin in a woman's system cause strong contraction of the uterus, thus aiding a return to its pre-pregnancy condition.
- Oxytocin release is vulnerable to conditioning and this assists a woman to want her baby in a biological way, consolidating the bonding process — when she sees or hears her baby, the milk begins to flow and the mother needs her baby to nurse at her breast. Similarly, oxytocin can be easily conditioned by negative inputs, so that in certain circumstances her milk will refuse to flow. The biological basis for this action ensures that a mother will not let down her milk for another child, thus ensuring survival of her own infant. This effect is of more significance in herd animals, where milk stealing by others may jeopardise natural offspring.

For a woman, the production of oxytocin during her reproductive life causes frequent rhythmical contractions of her uterus. These are rarely noticed, being similar to the wave-like contractions of other smooth muscles in her body. At times, particularly during her menstrual flow, these contractions become stronger and more noticeable, as a result of the hormonal cycle and a resultant increased sensitivity in the uterus.

During sexual intercourse, the release of oxytocin is responsible for strong contractions of the uterus, causing an 'in-sucking' action at the cervix, designed to speed sperm transport into the uterus. The trigger for oxytocin production comes from either nipple, clitoral or vaginal stimulation, and in particular the distension of the vagina by the erect penis. The resultant uterine contractions create orgasmic feelings which are pleasurable and thus encourage further sexual contacts. In addition, the nurturing behaviours caused by the flow of oxytocin are directed towards the partner, assisting in the formation of a close bond. Some of the physical effects of oxytocin release can also been seen during intercourse — a rise in skin temperature and the release of body odour that is individual in character, for example.

PREGNANCY

Once a woman has conceived, oxytocin plays a role in maintaining the pregnancy. The in-sucking action of the cervix during the regular contractions of the uterus (Braxton-Hicks contractions) serves to keep the cervix tightly closed. Should there be a change in the levels of the other pregnancy hormones, notably an increase in prostaglandins, then this in-sucking action may change, and the cervix may begin to open. Normally this occurs at the onset of labour where the balance of oestrogen and progesterone changes and the level of natural prostaglandin increases. This sets off a change in the reaction of the cervix to oxytocin, and instead of its presence causing an in-sucking action, it reverses and the cervix begins to open. It has been suggested that the sudden production of prostaglandins, for example, in response to an infection, may be a factor in altering the hormonal balance resulting in a changed sensitivity of the cervix to oxytocin, perhaps leading to a premature onset of labour. The complex role of oxytocin in preserving the pregnancy also explains the lack of success in initiating labour (using natural or artificial means) until the physical climate in the woman's body is primed for birth.

LABOUR — FIRST STAGE

Once labour has begun, the ebb and flow of oxytocin shapes the pattern of the contractions. The hormone is released as a result of pressure from the presenting part of the baby against the cervix. If the head becomes well applied, the contractions become regular and consistent. If the baby is breech, the soft buttocks may exert a less even pressure, leading to irregular, less powerful contractions. A baby presenting in a posterior position, with a deflexed head, will exert pressures initially on the pelvic bones, especially the sacrum, rather than the cervix, and many of these labours start very slowly, with much backache and inconsistent contractions.

Whilst the membranes remain intact, the pressure from the head against the cervix will be cushioned by the bag of forewaters. With a well positioned head, the pressure will be transferred effectively through the intact membranes and the contractions will be efficient, whilst the baby's head will be protected from undue direct pressure. Once the membranes have ruptured, which usually occurs at the time of transition or during the early part of second stage, the baby's head will come into direct contact with the surrounding tissues and heavy, intense and sustained contractions will result. These strong contractions may be designed to achieve rapid dilatation and a speedier conclusion to the birth process.

If the membranes rupture at the beginning of labour, perhaps before the establishment of the favourable hormonal environment necessary for the initiation of labour, some time may pass without any discernible labour contractions. Once conditions are right, contractions will begin in the usual way, sensitivity to oxytocin will increase and labour will start.

If the membranes are ruptured artificially once labour has started, the removal of the cushioning bag of forewaters will cause the baby's head to press directly on the cervix. This may result in sudden stimulation and strong, powerful contractions for both mother and baby. Fetal distress may be triggered by the increased compression of the baby's head, and the mother may request pain relief, since her endorphin level may not yet be high enough to compensate for increased pain.

TRANSITION

The last few centimetres of dilatation are usually referred to as the 'transition' phase of labour. The uterine contractions begin to change their effect, from pulling the cervix open, to pushing the baby down through the birth canal. The amniotic sac frequently ruptures at this time as a result of extra pressure on the membranes. This, in turn, leads to sustained contractions useful in achieving the final centimetres of dilatation. These heavier contractions, and the resultant pain, cause endorphin levels to rise in response. If the membranes are still intact, the forewaters may bulge through the cervix, beginning an early desire to push even though the cervix may not be fully dilated.

SECOND STAGE

There may be a lull between first and second stage when dilatation is complete, yet the baby has not begun its descent which starts the next phase of oxytocin production. As a result, the contractions may cease, and the mother and baby may gain a welcome rest period. Once the head does begin to descend, oxytocin is released in response to the opening out of the pelvic floor muscles as the head passes through together with distension of the vagina. This is similar to the flow of oxytocin caused by the extension of the vagina by the penis during lovemaking, although the larger size of the baby's head will provide a greater stimulus to oxytocin production, and the resultant contractions will be much stronger. Perhaps this explains why some women describe birth as orgasmic — they experience the same hormonal release in both cases and recognise the sensations during birth as being similar to orgasm during sexual intercourse.

When the baby's head reaches the perineum, there is a further stretching of muscle and tissue prior to crowning. Once again, there is a surge of oxytocin in response to this stretching, to maintain the mother's pushing urge and to ensure there is oxytocin in her body for a short period after the birth. It is thought that the release of oxytocin at this point may also ensure colostrum is available in the breasts, to encourage the baby to find the nipple.

THIRD STAGE

After the baby is born, the uterus continues to contract to assist the placenta to separate and be expelled. This task is aided by another flow of oxytocin, this time as a result of nipple stimulation. The nipples are very sensitive immediately after birth, as they usually are following orgasm, and any touch of the baby's mouth or tongue will be registered. Of course, very soon the baby will begin to suckle, but even the preparatory nuzzling and licking can stimulate oxytocin release in the mother's body. Once the baby latches on to the nipple and begins to suck, there is a powerful surge of oxytocin, necessary for the expulsion of the placenta and the avoidance of haemorrhage. The amount of oxytocin released at this time is probably greater than at any other time during the labour.

As well as assisting in the completion of third stage and preventing bleeding, the rush of oxytocin through the mother's body raises her skin temperature, so that the baby stays warm when nestled against her, skin to skin, and floods her with nurturing feelings for the baby. Thus oxytocin becomes an important element in the initial attachment process between mother and baby.

BREASTFEEDING

It is no accident that oxytocin is the primary hormone involved in milk production. Without it, the milk would not reach the baby, and the mother would get no reward for offering her breast to the baby. Each time the baby suckles, the stimulation of the nipple causes oxytocin to be secreted, which in turn, contracts the smooth muscle fibres surrounding the milk sacs in the breast causing the milk to flow. This is known as the milk ejection reflex. Oxytocin is thus responsible for the milk reaching the baby, the skin of the breast being warm and comforting and the mother's feelings of tenderness towards her baby. In addition, she also experiences pleasurable feelings that can be very sensual, even sexual — a just reward for the intimacy of breastfeeding. The frequent feeding patterns of the young baby result in the mother feeling protective and nurturing towards her baby accompanied by sensual rewards for herself and thus mother and babe become bound together in an exquisite relationship. This closeness excludes the father to some extent, and although this is often interpreted as a potential problem for their relationship, it is probably a mechanism designed to ensure the spacing of pregnancies and the mother's complete focus of attention on the baby during its early vulnerable months.

The oxytocin released during nursing also affects the other receptor sites in the mother's body, and she notices uterine contractions, designed to speedily return her uterus to its pre-pregnancy condition.

Much of the analysis and identification of the action of oxytocin was completed by early lactational physiologists such as Niles Newton and Walter Whittlestone. Newton was the first to describe the 'fetus ejection reflex' in which the body produces a surge of oxytocin in response to extreme fear at critical times during birth. Instead of inhibiting labour it has the reverse effect, producing one or two enormous contractions that result in an immediate arrival of the baby. More about this interesting phenomenon in a later section.

IN SUMMARY

FACTORS THAT INCREASE OXYTOCIN PRODUCTION

- Distension of the vagina
- Clitoral stimulation
- Pressure on the cervix, in the presence of prostaglandins, which increases the sensitivity of the cervix to oxytocin
- Distension of the pelvic floor muscles during second stage
- Stretching of the perineum during crowning
- Nipple stimulation

FACTORS WHICH INHIBIT OXYTOCIN PRODUCTION

Direct

- Fear or anxiety caused by:

    external factors — being moved during labour, unpleasant smell, strange people, noise, distractions, bright lights, feeling exposed etc.

    Internal factors — concerns about the baby's health, worry about perineal tearing, fear of pain etc.
- Anaesthetic injections (epidural, pudendal blocks, local anaesthetics), which numb the nerves at receptor sites necessary for the initiation of the Ferguson Reflex.
- Induction and augmentation, which flood the receptor sites with abnormally high levels of oxytocin, rendering them less sensitive to the physiologic doses produced by the body.
- Episiotomy, which reduces the stretching of the perineum, thus removing one triggering factor for oxytocin release.
- Separation of mother and baby at birth, leading to a lack of nipple stimulation necessary for maintaining oxytocin flow during the third stage of labour.

Indirect

- Beliefs and attitudes, which may lead to embarrassment, a powerful inhibitor of oxytocin.
- Memories, perhaps of past sexual abuse, which may remain subconscious (leading to an unexplained discomfort) or become conscious, leading to fear, embarrassment or anger.

Results of oxytocin inhibition

- Failure to achieve orgasm — perhaps leading to difficulties in long term relationships due to lack of oxytocin-initiated nurturing and caretaking behaviours between partners
- Slowing of labour — contractions are further apart
- Slower dilatation due to contractions of reduced strength
- Prolonged second stage of labour — due to little or no urge to push
- Increased likelihood of post-partum haemorrhage following birth
- Problems with breastfeeding due to a faulty milk ejection reflex.

Further reading

Lincoln D. 1974, 'Maternal hypothalamic control of labour', in *Progressive Brain Research*, vol. 41, Elsevier Scientific Pub Co, The Netherlands.

Newton N. 1971, 'The trebly sensuous woman', *Psychology Today*, July, pp. 68–71.

Newton N. 1978, 'The role of the oxytocin reflexes in three interpersonal reproductive acts: coitus, birth and breastfeeding', in *Clinical Psychoneuroendocrinology in Reproduction*, Academic Press, pp. 411–418.

Newton N. 1987, 'The fetus ejection reflex revisited', *Birth*, vol. 14, no. 2.

Odent M. 1984, *Birth Reborn*, Random House.

Odent M. 1987, 'The fetus ejection reflex', *Birth*, vol. 14, no. 2.

Whittlestone W. G. 'Obstetric practice and lactation: the inhibitory effects of large doses of oxytocin', personal communication.

Wiggins J. 1979, *Childbearing physiology, experience, needs*, CV Mosby.

Chapter 6

The pain of labour

When we are born, we arrive in the world equipped with innate and instinctive behaviours designed to ensure that we survive, to eventually reproduce and therefore perpetuate our species. The controlling centres for these essential behaviours are in the hypothalamic region of the brain, often called 'the ancient brain', and the instincts involved are implanted there very early in fetal life. Most of the time, the circumstances that fire off the 'flight or fight' mechanisms of survival will be different from those that encourage us to reproduce. During labour and birth, the two areas become interconnected since the mother and baby are very vulnerable at that time, and a successful outcome will depend on their safety and protection with no potentially life threatening situations disturbing the process. Should a threat arise, nature instigates a series of life-preserving reactions designed to increase the chances of survival. It is the interplay of these delicate mechanisms that dictates much of the physiology of labour and birth and which stimulates much of maternal behaviour at that time.

These behaviours are governed by the release of several hormones in a complex and automatic process. The main hormonal players in these events are oxytocin, endorphin and the catecholamines (adrenalin). We cannot physically control their release and turn them on and off at will. They are secreted automatically in response to perceived (apparent) and direct events detected by our bodies and give rise to instinctive reactions and innate responses.

The flow of labour, as we have seen, is controlled by oxytocin. This hormone is sensitive to adrenalin, which drives the survival behaviours. The role of endorphin is to protect the mother during labour from excessive pain, to raise her sensitivity to her body's needs and to enable her to labour more effectively.

The main symptoms of labour are contractions of the uterus and a varying level of pain. There is no doubt that parts of labour are painful for a woman. Very few women labour without some degree of pain, and therefore this universal experience must have a specific purpose, an integral role in the reproductive process. It seems likely that there are two main reasons for the presence of some pain during birth — one physical, the other psychological.

The primary reason concerns the need for a woman to know firstly that she is in labour, and secondly, how far she has progressed so she can judge the arrival time of the baby. This is important if she is to find a safe place in which to give birth, and to settle there in good time so that she and the baby are protected from possible harm. All animals either prepare or identify a special birth place and make their way there when they sense that birth is imminent. In addition, it is interesting to note that nocturnal animals give birth during the day and diurnal animals at night — a mechanism designed to ensure privacy from other members of the species and reduce the risk of disturbance by natural predators.

Contractions have a specific character according to the stage of labour and this provides the biofeedback mechanism that lets a woman judge her progress. The twinges and sporadic contractions of early labour announce the beginning of the birth process whilst the unmistakable power of contractions during transition indicate that the birth is approaching. Pushing contractions in second stage are a reliable sign that the birth is imminent. At each stage a woman reacts differently to these stimuli and an experienced midwife can often tell the rate of dilatation of the cervix from observation of the woman's reactions to her contractions, without the need for invasive internal examinations.

Women who have painless labours or precipitate births often find these very unpleasant or frightening experiences. Perhaps the signals of an impending birth (usually transition contractions) trigger innate fears for the safety of the baby, should it arrive before a protected birth place can be reached. The combination of having to manage huge contractions before the endorphins have had time to be released, the urgency of needing to find a safe birth place and the anxieties produced by the unexpected circumstances, could be expected to leave women reporting that short labours are extremely unpleasant.

The psychological advantages of experiencing pain in labour have often been mentioned by women. Accepting the powerful sensations created by the labouring uterus and riding with strong and sometimes painful contractions to produce the miracle of a baby, offers women unique opportunities for self-discovery and growth through mastery of this potentially life threatening situation. Submission to the all-consuming and overwhelming nature of birth and the weathering of the inherent pain of labour is an empowering process for a woman, and one which she should not be denied unless critical for her own well-being or that of her baby.

WHERE DOES THE PAIN COME FROM?

The basic pain messages received by the brain during labour stem from the stimulation of sensory nerves in the uterine muscle mass. The uterus contains sensory nerve endings that register sensations caused only by stretching and tearing. There are no specialised nerve endings that react to other stimuli such as cutting, application of heat, cold, pressure etc. Therefore the primary source of pain is the stretching of the cervix. The need for a clear signal in the unlikely event that the uterus was tearing is obvious, as this is a life threatening situation for the woman and her baby.

Other abdominal organs and tissues surrounding the uterus have additional sensory nerve fibres and may register a variety of sensations: pressure from the uterus and baby as the labour advances; pressure on a full bladder or bowel; pain from compression of nerves and bones caused by the position of the baby's head, etc. These additional discomforts can often be eased, and are peripheral to the pain of the actual birth process.

As labour gathers strength the nature of the contractions changes and the amount of pain registered by the woman increases. This provides a mechanism for assessing progress in labour. As the end of first stage nears, the contractions become very intense, closer together and much more painful. The mother enters the transition phase between first and second stage and involuntary changes in her behaviour occur. The pain is stronger because the contractions are longer and a greater stretch is being exerted on the cervix to open it the last few centimetres. Once the cervix is fully open, the baby begins to descend through the birth canal, and the sensations again change in nature. Pain is no longer initiated by the stretching cervix as this is fully open, but the mother may register pressure on tissues surrounding the vagina, or on the pelvic bones, if the baby is a tight fit.

If the cervix opens unevenly, cervical pain may still be felt even though the mother is apparently into second stage, indicated by her desire to push. If a woman finds pushing painful, especially if there are no signs of descent, the cervix may have dilated unevenly with an anterior lip that may be impeding progress. Appropriate measures must be taken to reduce pressure from the baby on this lip of cervix until it is fully retracted (this is best achieved by the mother assuming a knee-chest position).

In early second stage (the latent phase) the contractions can be mild, with few pushing urges. There may even be a complete break, allowing time for mother and baby to rest before beginning the work of birth. This rest period is more common in primiparous women. As momentum builds up, the pushing urges become more organised as the uterus undertakes the expulsion of the baby. As the baby descends through the birth canal, the pelvic floor muscles open out and the vagina unfolds to accommodate the baby on its journey towards birth. Pain from the stretching of the cervix is absent, but the opening of the pelvic floor muscles could be painful, unless they are completely relaxed. The vagina is capacious and unfolds easily. When the baby's head reaches the perineal tissues, they begin to stretch slowly. This causes the stinging 'rim of fire' sensation that heralds the baby's imminent arrival, usually passing in minutes as the baby's head crowns and is born.

The sources of pain described above are normally present in labour, and form an integral part of the process. The amount of pain a woman will register is modified by many factors, some physical and others psychological. Pain will be increased if a woman is frightened or anxious during labour, if she assumes uncomfortable positions (which place undue pressure on surrounding structures and tissues), if her baby is malpositioned (for example, presenting in the occipito-posterior position), or if there is some other mechanical problem such as cephalopelvic disproportion or a full bowel or bladder obstructing progress.

Such messages of extreme pain are diagnostic and encourage a woman to seek remedies to reduce the physical causes of her pain. Severe pain in second stage can indicate a tight fit between the baby and the pelvic bones, with extra pressure being felt on the sacrum or ischial spines. This situation is exacerbated by unphysiologic positions for birth, particularly semi-sitting, and a change of position may relieve the pain. Touching the perineum in second stage is also painful for the mother and should be avoided by caregivers.

Pain is an integral part of labour for almost all women, a fact acknowledged by the body's ability to produce its own pain modifying substances — endorphins — to assist women through the rigours of labour.

ENDORPHINS

Endorphins are natural substances similar to opiates in structure and effect that are produced in the brain stem, nerve endings, and even the placenta. They appear whenever the body is physically stressed beyond its normal limits. A common example of endorphin release, and one familiar to most people, is the 'jogger's high' that runners experience when reaching a level of physical stress beyond which they would not normally be able to continue. At this point the runner's body releases a surge of endorphins. As a result, the jogger gets his 'second wind' which allows him to keep on running.

There are three main effects of endorphins: they modify pain, create a sense of well-being, and alter perception of time and place. The behavioural effects of endorphins are quite noticeable, and can therefore be useful indicators of physical states. The behavioural effects of endorphins on labouring women are particularly helpful in assessing their progress and can be used diagnostically to assess of the normalcy of the labour.

In pregnancy, a woman's body undergoes a natural state of stress as it copes with the extra workload due to the requirements of the developing baby. Indeed, it has been said that being pregnant is a mild form of aerobic exercise due to the increased cardiac and respiratory output that is required by the mother. As pregnancy progresses, the level of endorphins gradually rises in response to this stress, and towards the end of pregnancy, she will have moderately raised levels much of the time. Many women report behavioural effects during the last few weeks of the pregnancy probably attributable to these increased endorphin levels: a feeling of well-being, of acceptance and readiness for the baby; broken sleep, a tendency to lie awake for hours; vivid dreams; noticeable maternal amnesia, etc.

Once labour begins in earnest, the endorphin level continues to rise. Early contractions are not usually more difficult to handle than the strains caused by daily activities. After some time in 'pre-labour' the contractions begin to strengthen, to a point where they are measurably stronger requiring concentration. Around this time, a woman begins to physically slow down to focus more directly on what is happening. It will be observed that the contractions are coming more regularly and somewhat closer together by now. This increase in tempo of the labour stimulates endorphin production, and its release is heralded by her change in behaviour. It is at this point that labour would be described as 'established'.

As labour progresses there is a need to contend with increasing fatigue and pain. The continued rise in endorphins helps the mother manage her labour. Her behaviour indicates that this process is occurring: she becomes withdrawn, more sedentary, rests between contractions, closes her eyes, and appears 'spaced out'. These signs are all proof that her endorphin levels are adequate for her needs and that the labour is progressing normally.

During the transition phase of labour, there is a physical upheaval as the uterus changes its action from opening the cervix to pushing the baby out. The contractions become quite painful, are closer together, and seem unremitting in their intensity. Endorphin production is at its highest at this point, assisting the mother to manage the pain, but also allowing her to focus inwardly. Many women become quite disoriented and the accompanying amnesic effect means that women often have difficulty remembering much of the detail of this part of labour after the baby is born.

Transition is often the point where women are suddenly confronted by overwhelming fears that they are unable to complete the birth, that they cannot cope and that, in extreme circumstances, they might die. It may be that the high levels of endorphins produce these hallucinations, and that overcoming this confrontation with life and death is important to the subsequent feeling of achievement reported by many women after birth. Little is known about the psychological effects of endorphins in labour, but their presence in normal labour probably serves an important psychological as well as physical purpose.

Once transition passes the contractions usually slow, become shorter and may even stop for a time. The high levels of endorphins engendered by the powerful transition contractions create a feeling of well being and help a woman to get her second wind. Even women who have had very long and arduous labours can experience this surge of energy at the beginning of second stage.

During second stage, endorphin levels remain high in response to the work of pushing. As soon as the baby is born, the effort of labour ceases and the woman experiences the characteristic euphoric state of high endorphin levels. She is elated, feels a sense of achievement, and is in a positive and receptive state, important for greeting her new baby.

It may well be that one of the most important reasons for endorphin production during labour is to ensure this optimal physical and emotional state immediately after the birth. From the baby's perspective, it is important that its mother is alert, welcoming and intensely interested in nurturing and protecting her newborn. This is vital for the baby's survival immediately after the birth and for the development of close bonds of attachment. A mother in a euphoric state is likely to fulfil these needs of the baby, who in turn, displays behaviour designed to appeal and attract attention in a positive way. Post-birth elation due to endorphins will not be present unless the endorphins have been stimulated into production earlier in labour as a response to the contractions. Therefore, experiencing labour together with its pain, may be essential precursors for the bonding behaviours necessary for ensuring survival of the infant.

Following the birth, the endorphin level in the body falls dramatically, and about two days after the birth has returned almost to pre-pregnancy levels. The 'third day blues' that many women experience are thought to be a reaction to the sudden withdrawal of endorphin she has had in her body (and to which she has become addicted) over the previous nine months. On the fourth and fifth day the levels of endorphin rise a little, and then gradually taper off, returning to pre-pregnant levels by around three weeks after the birth.

INHIBITION OF ENDORPHINS

PETHIDINE

Research has shown that giving the mother pethidine (meperidine) does not interfere with endorphin release during labour. Pethidine, a synthetic opiate, is chemically similar to naturally produced endorphin, and indeed some of the same behaviour associated with endorphin release can be observed following administration of pethidine. Pethidine, however, being synthetic and given in high dosages, produces side effects which can be serious for mother and baby. Further information on the side effects of all the medications used in labour can be found in *Preparing for Birth*.

EPIDURAL

The use of epidural anaesthesia in labour has a marked effect on endorphin production, and appears to remove it from the mother's system for the duration of the epidural. Since endorphin is produced in nerve endings as a response to physical stress, anaesthetising the nerve endings will limit endorphin production. Without the apparent physical stress on the body (the woman is now numb) the production of endorphins declines and this can be observed by a change in her behaviour. Following administration of an epidural, many women 'sober up' and the dreamy, 'spaced out' behaviour vanishes.

As the epidural begins to wear off many women find that the labour is more painful than before and request a top up. While anaesthetised, the labour will, it is hoped, have progressed and as sensation returns, the mother finds the contractions are much stronger. It will take some time for endorphins to be produced again in response to these heavier contractions, and meanwhile, the woman may experience considerable pain, and request help — a top up of the epidural.

If the epidural wears off as the mother goes into second stage, then she may not need the epidural topped up, since second stage is generally less painful. If, however, as a result of the epidural the baby requires a forceps delivery, then increasing the epidural cover is essential, to ensure adequate relaxation of her pelvic floor muscles and perineum.

Epidurals are often recommended for women who are having a long posterior labours. This suggestion is based on a desire to help a woman through the long and often painful hours of labour in these circumstances, promoted by the knowledge that an epidural is a usually reliable form of pain relief. However, women experiencing a posterior labour seem to produce especially high levels of endorphin in response to the heavier and more painful contractions, and it may be safer to leave pain management to a naturally produced substance than to administer an epidural, with its attendant side-effects and risks. With an epidural in place it is likely that the labour will slow down and the baby will find it more difficult to turn as a result of the loss of tone in the pelvic floor. She is more likely to need forceps, an episiotomy or a caesarean section.

Women with long posterior labours can be helped to weather labour without artificial pain relief, if attention is paid to ensuring that endorphin production is not inhibited. Endorphins can protect her from the additional pain caused by the baby's position, help her lose track of time, make her want to rest as much as possible, and provide her with energy in second stage. These women often feel especially elated after the birth and may not sleep for many hours. Their remarkable resilience and stamina in labour may be directly attributable to the powerful effects of endorphins.

NITROUS OXIDE

Little is known about the effects of nitrous oxide on endorphin production. Anecdotal evidence suggests that since nitrous oxide is generally used for a short period in labour, it does not seem to interfere with the mother's levels of endorphin. The effects of nitrous oxide, as well as other drugs, on endorphin production is a fertile avenue for research.

CATECHOLAMINES

When a person is frightened, fearful or in a potentially dangerous situation, the body automatically turns on survival behaviours, and releases hormones called catecholamines, commonly known as adrenalin and nor-adrenalin. These hormones are made in the brain, in the adrenal glands on top of the kidneys, in the nerve endings in the body, and in other locations. They act on nerve endings of the sympathetic nervous system, and produce what is commonly called the 'fight or flight' syndrome, a series of behaviours designed to effect a rescue from the source of danger.

We have probably all felt their effects at some time in our lives, and can recall a pounding heart, rapid breathing and a feeling of wanting to run away from the danger. Other symptoms of the syndrome are: an increase in blood sugar levels; a rise in blood pressure; a decrease of activity in the digestive system; a decrease of blood supply to the internal organs; cold clammy skin and dilated pupils. In other words, the body directs a flow of super oxygenated blood towards those parts of the body that are most useful in escaping from the danger — that is, the peripheral muscular system, the heart, the lungs, and the brain.

In labour, a woman finds that her body is subjected to a certain amount of stress, and as her labour builds in strength and she may breathe a little faster, her heart rate increases and her blood pressure may rise slightly. These are all normal responses of the body. If, however, she is subjected to additional distress from an external source that registers an alarm, her body will automatically release adrenalin to assist her. Poor labour environments, frightening comments from carers or uncomfortable positions, an increase in pain that raises anxiety, could all have this effect. Now she is in a situation where her body has registered a threat. It is important to note that the source of the threat may be obvious (external) such as hearing forceps being discussed or noticing consultations with the doctor going on behind her back, or it can be a perceived threat such as the pervasive smell of hospitals that may be a reminder of unpleasant past experiences. For some women the sense of threat may arise from psychological or emotional factors, for example, a fear that the baby will be handicapped, or when routine procedures become reminders of a sexual assault in the past.

In threatening circumstances, a woman feels a strong urge to seek safety for herself and her baby. The innate behaviours associated with survival and reproduction overlap at this point, therefore in addition to producing the normal survival behaviours associated with adrenalin production, reproductive behaviours must be slowed to avoid the baby arriving into a potentially dangerous situation.

The usual symptoms of adrenalin release will be noticed by caregivers: agitated and restless body movements; rapid breathing; direct eye contact with dilated pupils, shivering or cold extremities; raised blood pressure; rapid pulse. Mechanisms to slow labour are initiated:

- The levels of oxytocin fall, in proportion to the amount of adrenalin in the system. This has the effect of slowing the contractions, perhaps causing them to stop altogether, particularly if there is little oxytocin being released, for example, in the early part of labour. Once labour has become established, with moderately high levels of oxytocin flowing, the contractions may slow in response to adrenalin, but are unlikely to stop altogether.

- To prevent further dilatation of the cervix, and perhaps the untimely birth of the baby, adrenalin stimulates the circular fibres in the lower third of the uterus to contract, to halt further dilatation. This action has an important side effect — once these circular fibres begin contracting, they work directly against the action of the longitudinal and figure-of-eight muscle fibres in the uterus, thus setting up a pattern of opposed muscle action. The resultant tug-of-war within the uterine muscle layers causes considerable pain, and may suggest that the contractions are working normally. Often, the combination of apparently strong contractions coupled with a lack of dilatation is labelled 'failure to progress' or worse, 'inco-ordinate uterine action', when in fact the phenomenon is a perfect example of the body's ability to respond normally, given the circumstances. Many women have had their uterus labelled as inefficient when in reality it was working perfectly. The additional pain from this opposed muscle contraction can be very intense and further adds to a woman's fear, especially if she is told that these powerful contractions are not producing any dilatation. A request for pain relief is therefore likely.

- A further development of the normal action of adrenalin in re-organising the internal blood supply in frightening situations, is that the uterus finds itself contracting with reduced blood flow and therefore less oxygen. Contractions of the uterus, which is made up of smooth muscle fibres, are not normally painful, but if the blood flow is reduced, then the muscle will become hypoxic, and painful when contracting. This is similar to the contractions of the heart — not normally painful unless the blood supply is blocked, perhaps by occlusion of a coronary artery.

The appearance of catecholamines (adrenalin and nor-adrenalin) in labour has an impact on endorphin levels. Endorphin levels fall in response to the 'flight/fight' syndrome triggered by adrenalin, and will only rise again when the source of the disturbance is removed and the woman is able to gain her equilibrium. Since it takes time for endorphin production to be re-established, allowance must be made for this to happen, and for the labour to gather pace and progress. Therefore, a useful rule of thumb is to allow an hour before checking for progress in dilatation. In practice, a woman may need an hour or more in the shower or bath, for example, to reduce her adrenalin level and to allow endorphin production to resume.

THE FETUS EJECTION REFLEX

When a woman in heavy labour is confronted by a fear inducing situation, the labour may be so well established that it would be impossible to slow it down, and she may be so immobilised by the overwhelming nature of the contractions that 'fight or fight' is physically impossible. Given these circumstances, often present during transition or the last moments of second stage, the sudden appearance of a rush of adrenalin has the opposite effect on the woman's body and instead of slowing or postponing the birth, it speeds labour up, to enable the baby to be born immediately. The reason for this phenomena, first described by Niles Newton in 1963, is to effect rescue for the mother and baby from a potentially dangerous situation. Instead of being immobilised by heavy labour, it can be advantageous to have the baby born as quickly as possible, so the mother is free to stand and fight or carry her baby away.

Instead of the adrenalin inhibiting oxytocin it causes a surge, followed by one or two huge contractions and the precipitate birth of the baby.

The stimulus for the rush of adrenalin may be obvious (many babies have been born very quickly once forceps are produced) or more psychological in nature. During transition, many women are frightened by the strength and power of the contractions and express this fear verbally — 'I can't do this', 'Just get the baby out', 'I can't take any more of this'. Sometimes, even very negative comments may be heard — 'Just give me a caesarean', 'I want to die'. Perhaps this is the 'moment of truth' for many women, when they face the need to find the resources to survive the onslaught of a tumultuous transition. It may be very important to allow women to have the experience of conquering an overwhelming personal crisis, to promote confidence and self-esteem in the new mother. Allowing expression of her negative thoughts (which she may not remember afterwards anyway) may be necessary to allow her to face the fear and deal with it. Reassurance or distraction may not, perhaps, be desirable or beneficial in the long run.

ADRENALIN AND THE BABY

The baby also produces catecholamines in response to the stresses of labour. Normally, as the uterus contracts, there is a reduced blood flow to the placenta, and to counteract this, the placenta stores oxygenated blood in between contractions, to ensure the baby's continued supply. An additional measure is provided by the production of adrenalin by the baby. This has the effect of shunting the available blood to those parts of its body where it is most needed — the heart, the lungs, the brain. In this way the baby is able to function normally during labour. Adrenalin also mobilises energy stores in the baby's body which will help it survive the reduced blood flow.

In addition, it has been shown that the production of catecholamines (in particular, nor-adrenalin) by the baby during the labour better prepares it for healthy functioning after birth. The production of nor-adrenalin mobilises the brown fat in the baby's body to produce heat and help maintain temperature after birth, dilates the pupils to encourage the mother to make eye contact and increases blood sugar levels to provide energy.

If the mother produces excessive catecholamines in response to anxiety, fear or stress, the baby can suffer from a lack of oxygen due to the reduced blood supply to the mother's internal organs, including the placenta. In turn the baby will react by producing excessive adrenalin, increasing the possibility of fetal distress and perhaps contributing to respiratory distress and metabolic acidosis. Therefore, it is vital that all sources of anxiety for a woman in labour be kept to a minimum, and that every attempt is made to enable the mother to labour with her own hormonal system intact, and with as little intervention in the birth process as possible.

IN SUMMARY

The clinical effects of catecholamine release in labour:

PANIC BEHAVIOURS

- restlessness, agitation
- loud noise — shouting, yelling
- wild movements
- activity
- wide, staring eyes
- raised blood pressure
- slowing of contractions, perhaps cessation
- increased pain during contractions
- a pause in dilatation — labour stalls with no further progress

OFTEN DIAGNOSED AS

- 'not in labour' — e.g. when the labour stops on arrival at the hospital
- 'failure to progress'
- 'arrested labour'
- 'inco-ordinate uterine action'
- 'dystocia'

MORE ACCURATE DIAGNOSIS

- 'a natural response to a threatening situation'
- 'normal rescue behaviours'
- 'perfect hormonal interplay in the circumstances'

SUGGESTED COURSES OF ACTION

- Identify the source of fear or disturbance and remove it
- Provide privacy and a small, safe labour environment (toilet? shower? bath?)

- Avoid unnecessary procedures, especially internal examinations.
- Change the environment — another room, immersion in water.
- Dim the light, provide warmth and quiet.
- Personal source of music (earphones) to block frightening noises.
- Reduce numbers of attendants, beginning with unnecessary staff.
- Provide continuity of caregiver, especially the constant support of a sensitive midwife.
- Allow time for adrenalin to decrease and endorphins to reappear — at least an hour in the new conditions.
- Whisper, avoid eye contact and conversation.
- Try counselling — particularly useful for emotional and psychological blocks during labour.

IMPORTANT POINTS

- If the mother and baby show no signs of medical problems, there is no need to take medical action.
- Avoid using negative language and labels as they colour perceptions.
- Oxytocin drips should be used only as a last resort when everything else has been tried and given time to work.
- If it is impossible to provide a non-threatening environment or a feeling of safety and protection for the mother, she may need an epidural to compensate for her lack of endorphins and the resultant pain caused by the circumstances. The giving of epidurals should be regarded as an acknowledgment of the failure to provide an appropriate labour environment, not as a rescue remedy she automatically needs or deserves.

Further reading

Dick-Read G. 1953, *Childbirth Without Fear*, Harper & Row, New York.

Ferguson J. 1941, 'A study of the motility of the intact uterus at term', *Surgery Gynaecology and Obstetrics*, vol. 73, pp. 359–366.

ICEA Review 1980, *Endorphins and analgesia*, ICEA, Minneapolis, USA.

Inch S. 1982, *Birthrights*, Greenprint.

Lagercrantz H. & Slotkin T. 1986, 'The "Stress" of Being Born', *Scientific American*, April 1986, pp. 92–105.

Nichols F. & Humenick F. 1988, *Childbirth Education: Practice, Research and Theory*, Saunders International.

Odent M. 1992, *The Nature of Birth and Breastfeeding*, Bergin & Garvey, USA.

Simkin P. 1986, 'Stress pain and catecholamines in labour: Part 1 A review', *Birth*, vol. 13, no. 4.

Simkin P. 1989, 'Non-pharmacological methods of pain relief during labour' in *Effective Care in Pregnancy and Childbirth*, eds I. Chalmers, M. Enkin & M. Keirse, Oxford University Press, Oxford.

CHAPTER 7

PATTERNS OF LABOUR

BIRTH BEHAVIOURS

Women know how to give birth. A woman who is encouraged to be instinctive and to tune in to her body during labour can discover exactly what she needs to do to make labour easier for herself and the baby. It is sometimes argued that modern women have lost the 'art' of giving birth and that culture and beliefs have so over-ridden women's natural responses that they require direction and assistance to birth normally. This overlooks basic innate drives to reproduce, and reproduce successfully, common to all species, and the ability of endogenous endorphins to create the necessary introverted and uninhibited states that form the basis for instinctive behaviours. Successful birth is far too important in nature for its achievement to be left to chance or luck: inbuilt mechanisms guide the process towards a successful conclusion, and these can be accessed provided a woman is willing to explore her hidden capabilities, and if she is provided with an environment conducive to this exploration.

It is true that many women allow cultural values, fashion and personal beliefs to inhibit their innate abilities. It is also true that the current medicalisation of birth encourages women to forsake their own resources and embrace technology and external guidance during labour. The folly of this approach is only now being revealed through rigorous scientific studies. Meanwhile, many women have discovered, to their cost in physical and emotional terms, the inherent risks of tinkering with nature.

A basic belief in womens' ability to give birth, unassisted, is at the centre of the empowerment process. Caregivers need to use every opportunity presented by their clients to learn about the endless possibilities of normal birth and to reinforce their trust in, and reliance on the natural process as fundamentally correct, unless there are clear, unequivocal signs that the mother or baby need help.

It also must be understood that some babies are not meant to live. In the natural world, the weakest do not survive — an essential mechanism to ensure strong breeding stock and the health of the population as a whole. The modern desire of medicine to save all babies and to cure all ills is creating unrealistic expectations, and leaving parents with sometimes insurmountable problems. It is to be expected that some babies will die, and whilst this is regrettable and tragic for those concerned, it must be accepted as part of the fabric of life.

Having established these basic perspectives, we can explore birthing behaviours with an open mind.

It is possible to recognise the various stages of labour by just watching a woman's behaviour. Women display many adaptive responses during labour and individual patterns emerge as labour progresses and the mother responds to her own needs. There are some common threads amongst many observable behaviours and by becoming familiar with these and encouraging support people to look for these general signs, an idea of the stage of labour, the rate of progress and the mother's needs can be gauged.

FIRST STAGE

Many first labours begin quite slowly. Some may take days to establish, stopping and starting intermittently until eventually a regular pattern becomes established. Some women find their membranes break with few other signs. It may then take many hours for their contractions to begin, and scientific evidence suggests that it is wise to wait for 48 hours before attempting any intervention to speed up labour, unless there are clear indications of a problem. This will provide more than enough time for the majority of women, who will by then be experiencing regular contractions or have even given birth. The period of waiting would be less stressful if women and their caregivers understood that there are only two reliable signs of being in labour:

- noticeable contractions, and
- a regular, consistent pattern to the contractions.

It may take many hours of intermittent and sporadic contractions before such a pattern develops, and these preliminaries should be regarded as just that, and not true labour. Appreciating this would enable women to accept these as early warning signs, not actual labour and the risk of anxiety over the slowness of the labour would be eliminated. In addition, accepting womens' individuality regarding the way they start labour should discourage caregivers from intervening too soon.

Most women can cope fairly easily with the first three to four centimetres of dilatation by keeping busy with their normal activities, pausing when necessary to allow the contractions to pass. During this phase many women seem quite 'normal' and enjoy chatting with friends, watching television, reading a book, or generally passing the time completing household tasks. Contractions are often mild and occur at manageable intervals, although for some women the spacing can be quite close.

As labour develops, a change starts to take place. Beyond four to five centimetres the rate of dilatation starts to speed up, and the contractions become more intense, more business-like. This is a good sign, because it is not so much the space between contractions that counts, but the actual length and strength of the contractions themselves that indicate how well the body is working. Until the contractions are lasting about a minute, there is not sufficient strength or power in them to result in much cervical dilatation.

Once she enters this accelerated phase of labour the woman's behaviour reflects the increasing work that her body is doing, and endorphins begin to be released to help her manage the labour. The signs and symptoms of this release have already been described.

The most noticeable change in behaviour comes with the arrival of transition. Apart from common physical symptoms of shaking, nausea and vomiting, many women show a complete change in their mental state. It is at this time many express their fears about what is happening, feeling overwhelmed and out of control. Some loudly demand pain-killing drugs, others state quite simply that they're not going on, or wish to go home; some roundly abuse everybody within sight. All of these behaviours are natural reactions to the intense, strong contractions that are characteristic of transition. Her uterus is doing its hardest work at this time in achieving the last few centimetres of dilatation, and often at a very rapid rate.

As the name suggests, the uterus is also in a transitional state, changing its action from one of opening the cervix, to pushing the baby down the birth canal. This is often indicated by early signs of the mother's need to push. Any woman who shows a sudden change in personality or physical behaviours, should be suspected of being in this transitional phase, even if a recent assessment suggested she still had much dilatation to complete. Some women dilate very quickly once labour establishes, and behavioural signs are often more reliable than internal examinations as a measure of progress. This is particularly true of multiparous women.

PREMATURE URGE TO PUSH

In general, a woman's urge to push can be regarded as an indication that second stage is underway. If, however, there are no signs of the baby descending with these pushes, then further investigation is warranted. Frequently an anterior lip of cervix will be impeding progress, and remedies to alleviate this problem, such as side lying or knee/chest position will relieve pressure on the cervix and allow it to dilate. Entering a warm bath may also help, by creating buoyancy, reducing gravity and engendering a more relaxed state.

Sometimes pressure from a bulging bag of forewaters may be distending the pelvic floor muscles and triggering the pushing urge. This may be compounded by the position of the baby's head — when the chin is deflexed it can create, in effect, a larger diameter of the head which places extra strain on the pelvic floor muscles.

Panic can sometimes be initially interpreted as transitional behaviour, especially when a woman has just arrived at the hospital and the staff do not know her. It is easy in these circumstances to think that the mother must be almost ready to give birth, but after some time, with no signs of progress, examination often reveals little dilatation. When this happens, panic reducing measures must first be employed to calm the mother so she can begin to labour more effectively.

SECOND STAGE

Second stage is heralded by new behaviours. The turbulence of transition has usually passed, and the contractions slow or stop altogether for some time affording the mother a welcome break. Second stage contractions are usually shorter and more spaced apart. The surge of endorphins stimulated by transition produces a 'second wind' effect, and she becomes energised and focused as she begins to give birth.

As the pushing urge gradually builds, many women also become introspective as they decipher the new set of sensations they are experiencing. Many will close their eyes and withdraw to concentrate on the effort of giving birth. The sensation of the baby's head descending through the birth canal and the tight, burning feeling as the perineum begins to stretch, are internal signals, indicating to the mother that the baby is about to be born. Indeed, the pain from the stretching of the perineum is designed to help the woman hold back from pushing, to allow the perineum to stretch the final millimetres without tearing.

THIRD STAGE

The euphoric state created by endorphins and the alert, quiet state of the baby (elicited by the nor-adrenalin it has produced) work together to enhance bonding and attachment. The mother has eyes only for her baby and in turn, the baby seeks its mother's gaze and makes soft cooing noises to attract attention. The baby is capable of finding the nipple unaided if necessary, and attaching, to ensure early food and to cement the bond between them.

The mother, left to her own devices, will usually sit and hold her baby or lie down on one side with the baby nestled beside her. In an upright position there is little compression of the placental site, less chance of blood pooling and clotting, delaying placental separation, and full gravity to assist placental expulsion. This is best position for reducing the risk of haemorrhage, and for observing the amount of blood loss.

The cord is left until pulsations have ceased: it can then be cut at any time, perhaps after the placenta has been born.

IMPRINTING

Imprinting is a non-reversible behavioural response acquired early in life, which can be triggered later by certain stimuli or situations. Birth is one such sensitive time, and it is likely that experiences during birth could imprint behaviours in the baby which could influence their later lives. Little importance has been given to the potential impact of imprinting at birth, yet it may prove to be critical to our understanding of some adult behaviours.

Several papers have been released by Bertil Johansen and his team of Swedish researchers demonstrating a correlation between pre-natal exposure to pethidine and later opiate addiction, and nitrous oxide and amphetamine addiction in teenagers. The mechanism for these addictions is thought to be based on imprinting: that for some individuals exposure to these chemicals during labour and birth imprints a euphoric state which is craved many years later. This research is the first to show potential long term effects of nitrous oxide used in labour and suggests that imprinting may be a powerful influence, worthy of further investigation. It also opens up the possibility that other events experienced by the baby during birth may produce effects later in life — the potential for investigation in this area is enormous.

IN SUMMARY

A good midwife can tell what is happening to a woman in labour through close observation of her behaviour both during and between contractions. It is important that birthing behaviour be understood as unique and important, and a reliable measure of progress.

BEHAVIOURS COMMON IN THE PRE-LABOUR PERIOD

- 'nesting' — cleaning, tidying, spurts of energy
- intuitive feelings and recognition of subtle changes in her body
- may want additional sleep

EARLY LABOUR

- excitement, nervousness, anticipation
- restlessness, energy
- diarrhoea
- twinges and mild, inconsistent contractions
- rupture of membranes (about 20% of women), with or without immediate contractions
- mucous discharge
- walks around
- makes conversation
- makes eye contact
- unable to sleep
- eats and drinks as usual
- needs active companionship — conversation, distraction

ESTABLISHED LABOUR

- sits and rests between contractions
- avoids conversation and eye contact
- head rests on arms or pillow
- needs to rest her legs — begins to sink towards the floor
- more comfortable upright
- is thirsty but gradually loses appetite for food
- finds own comfortable position
- needs companionship that is unobtrusive and non-disruptive

- develops own breathing patterns
- changes her behaviour only when necessary — becomes more passive

Transition

- shaking and vomiting are common
- sudden change in behaviour patterns that were previously established
- personality changes — irrational comments
- feels out of control, unable to manage
- requests drugs
- restless, needs to move, try different comfort measures
- noise — yelling, even screaming
- rupture of membranes

Second stage

- 'second wind', spurt of energy
- feels calmer
- sense of purpose reappears
- intensely introverted
- grips and needs physical support
- drops towards the floor, bends and opens knees
- sounds change — grunts, pushing noises
- sudden need to empty the bowels
- rupture of membranes (if not already broken)

Third stage

- attention solely on the baby
- elation, feelings of surprise, satisfaction, amazement
- sits upright to better see and hold her baby
- waits to pick baby up — fondles the baby first
- gathers baby to the breast

The role of support people

By definition, I describe anyone who attends a woman in labour as a support person. Therefore the partner, friends, relatives, siblings midwife, doctor, childbirth educator, (whoever is present) are all people whose primary task is to support the woman in labour.

The support provided by these companions involves the creation of a safe place for birth with protection and privacy for the woman and a permissive, accepting atmosphere. It may or may not include direct physical touching of her body (massage etc.) or other close personal attention. Many women basically need companionship and a secure place in which to labour — their bodies will do the rest. It must be understood that there is nothing that can be done by anyone, including the mother, to shape the actions of the uterus — labour will unfold naturally in its own fashion. 'Assistance' often turns into intervention, and even massage, stroking, and the giving of advice may be interpreted by women as distracting during labour.

Being with a woman in labour can raise many feelings in companions and these need attention, to avoid emotional intrusions into the mother's personal space. Anxiety is a particularly contagious emotion and anyone who is feeling anxious at a birth will transmit these feelings to the woman, who is especially sensitive to any source of fear, whether it be her own or that of caregivers or companions. Many birth interventions, drugs and obstetric procedures have been forced on women because the caregiver was anxious, and not because the mother or her baby needed help. Many fathers find birth behaviour bewildering or even frightening and they may need support to help them manage their emotions. These issues need to be understood and recognised, so that when they occur they do not hinder a woman from achieving a normal labour and birth.

Potential disruptions to normal labour

Women labour in a myriad of ways, and respond to the forces of pregnancy, labour and birth with individual style. Given freedom to respond instinctively, women demonstrate a surprising array of adaptations and reactions during the birth process that can enhance our learning about normal physiology.

Given an understanding of the basic hormonal interactions during birth, it becomes possible to predict the kinds of influences that may disrupt labour.

Caution must be exercised in diagnosing the source of a problem for a particular woman in labour, since what may be frightening for one woman may be reassuring for another. For example, many women find the use of electronic fetal monitors to be dehumanising during birth and resent the intrusion of technology. Some, however, find the constant beep of the monitor a reassuring sound, signalling that their baby is safe and well during labour. Always check your own suspicions with the woman herself, to avoid making assumptions, perhaps based on your own personal experiences.

Apart from the factors, already discussed, that promote catecholamine production in labour, there are other ways that labour can be disturbed.

PROLONGED BREATH HOLDING IN SECOND STAGE

The most characteristic sign of second stage is a woman's involuntary urge to bear down. The pushing urge is intermittent, usually lasting no more than about 6 seconds, and may be observed one or more times during a contraction. The involuntary nature of the reflex is illustrated by a woman's inability to completely block the need to push — it is as hard to avoid pushing when the need arises as it is to avoid vomiting when necessary.

In the past, in an attempt to speed second stage, women were encouraged or exhorted to push as much as possible during second stage, from the moment that full dilatation was confirmed. The rush to get the baby born highlighted the anxiety of the attendants, and the poor condition of many babies born following these enforced maternal behaviours, was used as a justification for their use. Therefore, any discussion on the nature of the pushing urge in labour will benefit from an understanding, not only of the way the pushing urge is triggered in the body, but also of why prolonged breath holding and over-enthusiastic pushing can be deleterious to both mother and baby.

If a woman holds her breath for extended periods in second stage then both she and the baby can suffer from exhaustion and distress. Much fetal distress is iatrogenic, and is caused by inappropriate actions by attendants, such as:

- Encouraging immediate pushing as soon as it is established that the cervix is fully dilated, ignoring any rest period that develops between transition and second stage.

  Result: The mother and baby have no recovery time between the stages of labour. Dips in the fetal heart rate are common as a response to transition and are an indication that the baby needs to rest before the second stage contractions become established. The mother, too, needs time to gather her energy, develop her second wind and regain her equilibrium.

- Organising the woman into a recumbent position. This is often done to allow better access by caregivers in case problems develop. It also enables the perineum to be clearly viewed, important if further manoeuvres such as forceps or vacuum extraction are to be used in the event of a delay, or if an episiotomy is to be cut to speed up progress.

Result: The weight of the uterus presses on the inferior vena cava, with the potential of slowing venous return to the heart and therefore cardiac output, resulting in less blood circulating to the placenta. The baby will still follow the curve of the sacrum as it progresses down the birth canal; however, this mechanism will direct the head upwards against gravity. This in turn, slows progress, as the head tends to slip back between contractions. The woman will have to work extra hard to maintain progress and in addition she becomes a patient, more likely to be passively accepting of the situation.

Lying on her back may exacerbate the feelings of being out of control that she felt during transition, though instead of being a normal reaction to the labour, they are now generated by a feeling of helplessness precipitated by her passive, 'patient' position. Being stranded and vulnerable, with the genital area exposed, may also revive memories of sexual abuse for some, and create feelings of panic in others.

- Exhorting the woman to push, for as long as possible, with her chin forward on her chest and lungs full of air, whilst the contraction remains in force. Strong eye contact and firm direction from one or more caregivers is often used to encourage compliance.

  Result: Filling the lungs with a large volume of air then trapping it there through blocking of the diaphragm can create a sufficiently high pressure within the chest cavity to slow the flow of blood back to the heart. This in turn results in reduced blood flow to the placenta, and therefore to the baby. In addition, by holding the breath for a long time, perhaps up to fifteen seconds, the normal oxygen exchange will not occur in the lungs, and the blood that does flow through to the baby will be less oxygenated than it should be. Both of these conditions, the reduced blood flow and a reduced oxygen level, can lead to the baby's becoming distressed. Paradoxically, this prolonged breath holding also makes second stage longer. To try to make the body expel the baby by pushing when the uterus is not actively involved only serves to exhaust the mother and reduce her ability to work effectively with the normal pushing urges when they do occur.

- If there are indications that the baby is becoming distressed, or if the caregivers are anxious to get the baby born as quickly as possible, insisting that the mother doubles her efforts. Cutting an episiotomy will speed progress by avoiding the need to wait for the tissues to stretch. Forceps, to lift the baby over the perineum, are also often employed at his point, especially if it is judged that the mother's efforts are insufficient, or that she is exhausted.

Result: The conditions of low oxygenation of the blood, a reduced blood flow to the baby and maternal exhaustion will be exacerbated. The woman may feel inadequate at getting her baby born, and disappointed at her apparent inability to achieve birth without assistance. She may also receive an unnecessary episiotomy or forceps lift-out, neither of which she may have wanted or needed, had second stage been managed physiologically.

- When the baby is born, especially if it is slow to breathe, very mucousy, and unresponsive, feeling pleased at having rescued the baby, using the baby's condition to justify these actions.

Result: The continuation of an unscientific approach to second stage management, with serious side-effects for mothers and babies.

It is easy to see how fetal and maternal distress can be precipitated through the application of unphysiologic pushing techniques. The research establishing these links between inappropriate physical behaviour and poor fetal outcomes was described by Dr Roberto Caldeyro-Barcia in the 1970s and published in 1978. As President of the International Federation of Obstetricians and Gynaecologists during those years, the problems of second stage management were widely publicised, yet still these behaviours persist.

MATERNAL AND FETAL DISTRESS

There are several measures than can be taken to avoid these problems. Firstly, it must be remembered that the uterus is designed to expel the baby whether or not the mother contributes by pushing. This mechanism is designed to ensure the baby has a chance of being born, should the mother be unable to assist (for example, if she was unconscious). Today, this mechanism can be seen in women who have epidurals, and no urge or ability to push. The uterus forces the baby through the birth canal of its own accord, with the mother playing no part in its progress.

Secondly, we need to trust that a woman's body, having accomplished the growth and development of the baby thus far, knows how to get the baby safely born. Having invested energy to grow a baby, nature is not likely to jeopardise the baby's survival through naturally risky birth mechanisms. Therefore we must trust the woman and her instincts, and recognise that given the right conditions, she is capable of finding a safe passage for her baby.

IN SUMMARY

Specific actions that can be taken by the caregivers to avoid fetal and maternal distress in second stage:

- Use physical indicators such as a pushing urge, signs of fetal descent, anal pouting, changes in sounds, the need to be upright, the opening of the knees etc. as signs that second stage has begun. Full dilatation means that first stage is complete. Second stage may take time to become established, perhaps after an extended rest period.

- Place no arbitrary time limits on second stage. Provided that there are signs of progress, and both mother and baby are well, there is no need to hurry.

- Provide a safe, private, permissive environment where the woman can choose an appropriate position. Discourage her from getting on the bed, which may initiate the instinct to lie down (associated with beds). Keeping her off the bed will automatically ensure that she stays on her own feet and adopts an upright stance.

- Give her no directions. Avoid instructions, eye contact, conversation, confrontation, and unnecessary handling, especially of her perineum, which will be tender and sensitive as it stretches.

- Give her the responsibility for getting the baby born. This can be achieved by quietly encouraging her to work with her own body, to push only as necessary, and to take her time to work with her baby to achieve a gentle birth.

PERINEAL TRAUMA

The measures described above will not only encourage a safe arrival of the baby but will also serve to protect the woman's perineum from unnecessary damage. In the past, many episiotomies were cut in the mistaken belief that a neat cut healed faster, was more comfortable, and prevented uncontrolled tears. Scientific analysis of episiotomy has disproved these claims. Women, however, do want to avoid damage to the perineum and the following suggestions may help:

FOR THE WOMAN

- Choose your caregiver wisely. A midwife is much less likely to perform an episiotomy than an obstetrician. Ask about the personal episiotomy rate of the chosen caregiver, and change practitioners if necessary.
- Perineal massage during the last weeks of pregnancy may help to soften the tissues and reduce the likelihood of tears. The main purpose of this massage is to help women become familiar with their anatomy and accustomed to stretching and burning sensations common in second stage.

IN SECOND STAGE

- Choose a comfortable, efficient position.
- Allow time — don't be rushed into giving birth.
- Only push as much as the body indicates is necessary. Big babies and first babies require more effort than small babies, premature infants, twins, and subsequent babies.
- Keep your eyes and ears closed, to allow you to concentrate on the message from within your body. Try to block out distracting instructions from others.
- Avoid looking in a mirror — it can be confusing and takes your focus out of your body.
- If you are unsure about what is happening, try touching the baby's head in your vagina. This often clarifies the situation.
- Know that between you and the baby, a way out will be found. Take time to savour the process!

FOR THE CAREGIVER

- Protect the woman's right to choose her own position for birth. Be an advocate for her at this time.
- Avoid giving instructions. Commenting that she will know what to do and should take her time, may be helpful.
- Avoid touching the perineum — it is sensitive and tender and touching this area will cause acute pain. A warm, wet compress may be helpful instead.
- Avoid injecting local anaesthetic, in case an episiotomy is to be cut. Spongy tissues do not stretch well.
- Don't make eye contact — encourage her to close her eyes to stay focused on her task.

- Take your time — the baby will come when it is ready. Avoid manipulating the baby, especially to deliver the shoulders. Be ready to catch instead.

Time limits

Imposing time limits on labouring women is not only unscientific, but detrimental to her psychological and emotional state. As long as there is progress, and no sign of medical problems for either mother or baby, there is no justification for setting arbitrary limits to the length of labour, especially in second stage.

Some women take many hours (even days) of early pre-labour contractions before establishing productive labour, and it has often been noted that for the majority of women, once they finally 'get going' in labour, they seem to take roughly the same time — perhaps around 12 hours for a first baby and less for subsequent children. Of course, there are variations, and it may be that extended labours in some cases reflect disturbances to oxytocin production or the presence of adrenalin.

Pre-labour rupture of membranes poses a particular problem. It is quite common for a woman to find her membranes have ruptured, with no other signs of labour. This situation can extend for many hours, even days. The scientific evidence suggests that 48 hours is a reasonable time to wait before initiating labour artificially, and that the risk of infection to the baby is almost non-existent, provided that nothing is inserted into the vagina.

A problem arises when caregivers, often practising according to habit rather than on scientific grounds, impose a time limit then stimulate labour artificially. The woman waits for further signs of labour, with a clock ticking away, and as the time passes her anxiety increases, especially if she wished to avoid an induction. As a result it is likely that her adrenalin level will be high enough to completely negate any oxytocin that might be produced. She is often coerced into accepting an induction through threats of infection and dire consequences for the baby, but the greatest risk may come from the induction itself, with its resulting well-known cascade of intervention.

Women who begin labour in this way need a supportive environment which is unlikely to produce adrenalin. Sleeping, eating and regular daily activities are a must, together with some counselling to allow the expression of fears and concerns. Almost every women, in these circumstances, will begin labour within 48 hours of the membranes rupturing, a few will take longer. The baby's heartbeat can be checked (to allay the caregiver's anxiety) and the mother could be given prophylactic antibiotics after some hours, if potential infection is a concern.

In second stage, the application of rigid time frames on labour has had deleterious results, described above in the section on fetal distress. Again, as long as there is progress and mother and baby are well, it may be more important to let the baby make a slow and measured descent through the birth canal than a forced exit caused by unnatural maternal behaviours. Some babies, being larger, will take longer. Others, especially smaller or premature babies are easy to birth. It is a matter of allowing the mother and baby to work together as a team to negotiate the most appropriate journey.

The hormone oxytocin is especially sensitive to inhibition, as we have seen, and since birth is an innately sexual event, imposing time limits on this sexual act is as inhibiting for a woman in labour as it would be if she was trying to make passionate love with a partner with a stopwatch ticking towards a time limit (and the threat of 'assistance' if satisfaction is not achieved within the given time frame).

INTERVENTIONS DURING LABOUR AND BIRTH

Giving drugs in labour or applying obstetric interventions will undoubtedly disturb the normal flow of birth hormones. Any procedure, treatment or examination, however, has the potential to disrupt the natural behaviours of labour and impose new conditions on the mother. Possible inclusions on this list of stressors are:

- being moved from place to place during labour,
- being moved from the chosen birth place,
- giving birth in hospital,
- being asked to change out of own clothes,
- being asked to lie down on a bed for a physical examination,
- internal vaginal examinations,
- constant checking of the baby's heartbeat,
- attachment of machines (e.g. electronic fetal monitor),
- being left alone in a strange place,
- visits by strange staff during labour,
- change of staff during labour,
- lack of privacy,
- rupturing of membranes,
- setting up of drips,
- restrictions on movements.

Some of these disruptions, for example, checking the baby's heart beat, may be considered essential by staff. This assumption may be questionable for a woman who is labouring well (indicated by the presence of endorphins and the absence of adrenalin) since in this case it is likely that the baby will be doing well too. Whenever the mother needs to be approached to have the fetal heart checked, it should be done in the least disruptive way possible.

The need for frequent vaginal examinations certainly needs to be challenged. Each time an internal is performed the risk of infection rises. The woman is subjected to an unpleasant and often painful experience. Many caregivers have not learned how to carry out the procedure with the woman in any other position than recumbent on a bed, which forces her to adapt to the caregiver's lack of skill. Moving from place to place, even from a mat on the floor to a nearby bed, can cause an interruption in the flow of labour.

Women who have suffered some form of sexual abuse in their life (estimated at 25% of the adult Australian female population, for example) may find many procedures and conditions imposed during labour extremely threatening. Being asked to lie down in a submissive position may be confronting, and elicit painful memories. Internal examinations may be intolerable for these women. Any handling of their bodies, particularly in the genital area, may cause acute anxiety and distress. Victims of sexual abuse are unlikely to reveal their history to caregivers, but their plight may be suspected by the empathetic midwife. Every woman should therefore be regarded as a possible victim and treated with respect, gentleness and reverence in conditions that provide privacy and protection during labour and birth. Counselling is often this woman's primary need, not invasive, insensitive procedures applied because of 'the protocols'.

The effect of pain killing drugs in labour on endorphin production has already been described. All drugs have an effect, not only on the woman, but on the baby as well, and sometimes lead to interventions for the sake of the baby. The unpredictable effects of drugs on women and babies during labour is a major problem, and no safe levels can be assumed. The effect on the baby may last long after labour, with noticeable changes in the baby's reactions for days following birth, particularly following pethidine.

Before considering any intervention in birth, whether it be asking a woman to get on a bed, seeking permission to insert a drip, rupturing her membranes, moving her to another room, altering her position, subjecting her to an internal examination, caregivers should ask themselves: 'Is this really necessary?'. Often, the answer will be 'no' and the woman can be spared the discomfort and disruption of the procedure. Many procedures are performed as routine measures without adequate assessment of their need, or scientific proof of their safety or efficacy.

The 'cascade of intervention' has been well documented in the professional literature, yet it still persists. Perhaps if women understood the likely ramifications of interventions they would be better equipped to challenge the necessity of many proposed treatments. Activities that explore informed consent are described in Part 3.

DEALING WITH GRIEF

Many interventions in otherwise normal labour are performed 'just in case' something goes wrong at a later stage. Thus the fetal monitor is attached in case the baby's heart beat should slow or stop during labour; the drip line is inserted to avoid dehydration; the membranes are ruptured in case the meconium is stained; the bed is used for second stage to be ready for performing an episiotomy or forceps delivery.

This need to be pro-active is typical of the medical approach to birth and the necessity to be seen to be doing something, but it may also exemplify evasive actions brought on by unresolved grief from earlier professional disasters. Every caregiver must make a mistake on occasion, but acknowledging this can be difficult for the person concerned as well as for colleagues. Unless these griefs are resolved, lasting effects can colour behaviours for many years. The needs of parents in tragic circumstances are now better understood, and support and counselling services are usually provided to help them deal with their loss. Similar help should be available for staff in maternity units just as it is for workers in other personally stressful jobs, such as the fire brigade, the police service, the armed forces and the emergency services. Post traumatic stress is also well recognised for health professionals working in other areas of medicine such as cardiac units, cancer wards and palliative care, where death of clients is accepted, even expected. If maternity staff were able to call on appropriate counselling services when a disaster occurred in their unit, perhaps fewer obstetric interventions may be instituted in the mistaken belief that they will prevent future catastrophes.

THE BABY'S ROLE

Many women think that labour is solely their work, and are unaware that the baby is an active participant as well. It is the baby who indicates that its systems are sufficiently mature for independent life and that it is ready to be born. When ready, it signals to the mother using hormonal messengers. The mother's body then begins to prepare for birth and she seeks the right conditions so the labour can proceed safely. Much of this preparation goes unnoticed by the mother, but she may note signs that her labour is imminent, and that the pregnancy is drawing to a close. In those last weeks she will notice that her body is responding to the baby's message and is preparing for birth — the cervix softens, she has an increased vaginal discharge and perhaps a mucous show and the baby generally settles low into the pelvis. She becomes calmer and more introspective as she readies herself for the work that is about to begin. The baby usually becomes quieter as well, as if preparing itself for the effort of being born. The mother will choose a time to go into labour when her body feels calm, and her surroundings feel safe, often at night.

Once labour begins, the baby needs to wriggle itself into a good position, to find the way through the pelvis and birth canal to the outside world. For some babies this process will take quite some time, especially if the head is presenting initially in a posterior position. In this case, the baby may need many hours of gradual guidance by the muscles of the mother's pelvic floor and the shape of the pelvic bones gradually to turn round into a more favourable position for the birth.

The weight of the baby, assisted by gravity, ensures a steady pressure on the cervix during labour, especially if the mother is upright, and ensures that the Ferguson Reflex stimulates the release of oxytocin.

In second stage, the bones of the baby's skull can over-ride, to create a smaller diameter, thus easing the passage of the head through the pelvis. This clever design complements the mother's ability to open out her pelvic bones through suitable positioning. Being upright also ensures that gravity again aids the baby's descent through the birth canal.

Many mothers are surprised that the baby keeps kicking and moving around in the uterus during the birth process. The baby can use the top of the uterus as a springboard, and by pushing with its feet can help itself to dive down through the pelvis and birth canal. Sometimes these kicks of the baby are more disturbing for the mother than the actual contractions, but a baby kicking during labour is an indication of a healthy response to the stress of birth.

Many women find it helpful to talk to their babies during the labour, and to visualise the baby descending and emerging into their arms. This is a very natural progression from talking to the baby during the pregnancy, and it often helps women to focus on the activity within their body when they can make this kind of mental and physical connection with the baby during labour.

Babies born following normal labours, where no intervention has been necessary, are usually very quiet and alert. They open their eyes, and have the ability to control their body temperature. They are also better equipped to breathe spontaneously, the liquid in their lungs is more readily absorbed and the stores of glycogen in their liver are released to give them extra energy. The brown fat in the shoulder area is also mobilised to provide heat energy for the baby. These responses stem from the production of nor-adrenalin by the baby as a reaction to the stress of birth, and are important for extra-uterine adaptation. Any intervention in the labouring process has the potential to affect the baby and may reduce its capacity for normal functioning after birth.

FURTHER READING

Bennett A., Etherington W. & Hewson D. 1992, *Childbirth Choices*, Penguin.

Caldeyro-Barcia R. 1979, 'The influence of maternal bearing-down efforts during second stage on fetal well-being', *Birth & the Family Journal*, vol. 6, no. 1.

Caldeyro-Barcia R. 1979, 'The influence of maternal position on time of spontaneous rupture of the membranes, progress in labour and fetal head compression', *Birth & the Family Journal*, vol. 6, no. 1.

Crowther C., Enkin M., Kierse J. & Brown I. 1989, 'Monitoring the progress of labour' in *Effective Care in Pregnancy and Childbirth*, eds I. Chalmers, M. Enkin & M. Keirse, Oxford University Press, Oxford.

Davis E. 1987, *Heart and Hands*, Celestial Arts, California.

Flint C. 1986, *Sensitive Midwifery*, Butterworth-Heinemann.

Gaskin I. 1977, *Spiritual Midwifery*, The Book Publishing Company, USA.

Grant J. & Kierse M. 1989, 'Prelabour rupture of the membranes at term' in *Effective Care in Pregnancy and Childbirth*, eds I. Chalmers, M. Enkin & M. Keirse, Oxford University Press, Oxford.

Jacobson B., Eklund G., Hamberger L., Linnarsson D., Sedvall G. & Valverius M. 1987, 'Perinatal origin of adult self-destructive behaviour', *Acta Psychiatr Scand*, vol. 76, pp. 364–371.

Jocobson B., Nyberg K., Eklund G., Bygdeman M. & Rydberg U. 1988, 'Obstetric pain medication and eventual adult amphetamine addiction in offspring', *Acta Obstet Gynecol Scand*, vol. 67, pp. 677–682.

Jacobson B., Nyberg K., Gronbladh L., Eklund G., Bygdeman M. & Rydberg U. 1990, 'Opiate addiction in adult offspring through possible imprinting after obstetric treatment', *BMJ*, vol. 301, 10 November, pp. 1067–1070.

Kierse M., Ohlsson A., Treffers P. & Kanhai H. 1989, 'Prelabour rupture of the membranes preterm' in *Effective Care in Pregnancy and Childbirth*, eds I. Chalmers, M. Enkin & M. Keirse, Oxford University Press, Oxford.

Limburg A. & Smulders B. 1992, *Women Giving Birth*, Celestial Arts, California.

Odent M. 1990, *Water and Sexuality*, Penguin.

Simkin P. & Kitzinger S. 1990, *Episiotomy and the Second Stage of Labour*, Penny-press, USA.

Sleep J., Roberts J. & Chalmers I. 1989, 'Care during the second stage of labour' in *Effective Care in Pregnancy and Childbirth*, eds I. Chalmers, M. Enkin & M. Keirse, Oxford University Press, Oxford.

PART THREE

TEACHING ACTIVITIES FOR CLASSES

Chapter 8

Selecting teaching activities

Presenting exciting and effective pre-natal sessions involves more than luck or the possession of a vast repertoire of games that can be packed into every available minute. Running successful groups involves planning and careful selection of appropriate teaching strategies which are varied according to the group's needs.

There are a multitude of activities, exercises, games and teaching strategies that can be used in pre-natal classes. Enlivening the class through the use of a well-planned activity can have lots of benefits: participants are involved in the learning; they make social contacts with each other; it varies the presentation; the focus is taken off the leader; the group takes some responsibility for the learning; the learning is more effective.

When selecting activities, consideration must be given to:

- the size of the group,
- their learning styles,
- whether they like joining in or prefer passive participation,
- their level of education,
- the time available for completion of the activity,
- appropriate timing of the activity within the program,
- the number of participants in the group,
- the energy level in the group,
- the space available,
- the equipment needed,
- possible outcomes or reactions in the group to the activity,
- whether the activity will meet the set objectives for the topic.

This last consideration is most important. You will need to decide whether the activity you have selected is likely to meet your teaching objectives for the topic, and whether this activity is more suitable than others and appropriate for the group. You will also need to have a clear evaluation process, so that you can measure the success of the activity in meeting your stated objectives.

FOCUS ON SKILLS, MORE THAN KNOWLEDGE

In making the transition to parenthood, people will find that skills are more useful in the long run than knowledge alone. Confronted with a baby who cries at night, it may not be enough to know that something is wrong, it may be much more useful to know how to go about assessing the possible causes and how to develop strategies for managing the stress caused by the situation. The focus in pre-natal classes is changing, away from the giving of advice, the emphasis on information and the lectures on theoretical knowledge, towards the development of clearly defined skills that will be useful for new parents. Therefore, when choosing your class activities, select ones that are based on a skill, rather than ones that are purely for 'fun'. Parents will find these skills useful:

- the ability to solve problems (including gathering information, identifying choices, prioritising, making decisions)
- strategies for the management of stress
- the identification and use of personal resources (including instincts and feelings)
- the ability to find and utilise outside resources (how to consult 'experts', finding information etc.)
- the ability to be flexible in handling situations, seeing other people's points of view, negotiating alternatives, confronting important personal issues
- identifying personal limitations (including recognising crisis situations)
- the ability to take responsibility.

Your teaching objectives can be developed with a clear statement of purpose that focuses on the skills to be gained by parents through participation. Parents can be asked to 'identify choices', 'propose solutions', 'devise strategies' and 'list alternatives' as an integral part of an exercise. In this way, skills can be clearly described and the group's level of achievement in developing them can be noted.

It will be helpful to explain to your group your intention to focus on these skills. Many people come to classes expecting that you, as the teacher, will give information in much the same way as they have experienced in other learning situations. If you take some time to explain that the acquisition of factual information is only partly useful, and that knowing how to apply it is more practical, most adults will quickly understand and appreciate that you want to involve them directly in developing skills that they can apply in all areas of their future parenting.

The basic needs of adult learning have been described in Part 1 of this book. With these needs in mind, select class activities for their appeal to adult learning styles. Try to choose exercises and activities that involve the senses. Remember to introduce and summarise each activity for the linear learners and also those who need to understand the relevance of the activity to the bigger picture of overall goals.

PRESENTING TO YOUR GROUP

Introduce each activity carefully. Explain its purpose and the process, checking that your message has been understood. Once the activity begins, watch for individual and group reactions and clarify or repeat instructions if necessary. For example, if one small group is apparently puzzled by the process, go over the activity and explain what they are to do, using a different description. Check again that the process is understood.

When the activity is completed, mentally assess the group's reactions.

- Did it work?
- Were the objectives met?
- What comments do they make about the usefulness of the exercise?
- Did anyone have a specific reaction to the exercise? What triggered the reaction?
- Did the group enjoy participating?
- Did the activity run smoothly?
- Was there anything that could have been done to make it clearer?
- Is there a need for follow up in any area, as a result of this activity?
- Would I do anything differently another time?

Any unfinished business will need further attention, either immediately, or perhaps later, if individuals are involved.

TEACHING IDEAS

The activities that follow are intended to provide a selection of possible exercises for classes. Some, such as learning about the pelvis, are designed to assist in the development of a theoretical framework for the other activities that follow. Others are useful for developing social networks and enhancing group dynamics. Many are geared for the development of specific parenting skills. Many of these activities can be considered 'generic' in that the process remains the same, but the subject matter can be changed.

All can be considered as possibilities, to be used appropriately. These are just a selection of possible teaching strategies that can be incorporated into your teaching format. Others you can develop yourself, using this manual as a guide, or they can be gleaned from other teaching manuals. Some potential sources of ideas are listed at the end of this chapter.

I have included aims for each activity. You will need to develop specific learning and teaching objectives, so you are clear about how the activity will be presented, and what you want your clients to gain from their participation. I also want you to practise preparing objectives!

INTRODUCTION AND WARM UP GAMES

AIMS

✓ To provide opportunities for group interaction.
✓ To encourage networking and the formation of social support groups.
✓ To foster group dynamics.

INTRODUCE A PARTNER

Each member of the group finds someone they don't know, talks to them for a few minutes and then introduces them to the group. Partners can either be selected at random (turn to the person sitting beside you, not your partner) or teamed up (perhaps by selecting cards labelled 'knife' and 'fork', 'cup' and 'saucer', 'paper' and 'pencil', 'fish' and 'chips' etc. then finding the appropriate pair). There are many ways to mix up groups in this way.

CIRCLE NAME GAME

Everyone thinks of an adjective to link with their christian name, using the same initial. In turn, around the circle, participants introduce the people who came before them, with their adjective, starting with the first person, and putting themselves last. This may seem daunting, but is made easier in large groups by the fact that all the names will be heard many times as they are repeated by each person in turn.

BALL THROW

To consolidate and check that the names are now familiar to the group, a soft ball is tossed amongst the group, with the person throwing the ball calling out the name of the person who is to catch the ball. This continues until everyone is comfortable with the names.

For more ideas, check the resource list at the end of this chapter.

POINTS TO WATCH

☛ You may need to use an introduction game at the beginning of several classes to ensure that everyone knows the names.
☛ Take care to choose an activity that is appropriate for your group.
☛ Obtain permission from the group before handing out names and addresses, to protect their privacy.

IDENTIFYING GROUP MEMBERS' NEEDS

WHY ARE WE HERE?

AIMS

✓ To invite participants to state their reasons for attending the group.
✓ To identify individual needs of group members.
✓ To assist in the establishment of a teaching agenda.

PROCESS

In pairs, group members discuss their reasons for attending the class. Each person reports their partner's comments back to the group.

VARIATIONS

- Individual comments can be added to a large sheet of paper which is circulated.
- Members can add comments to a 'graffiti sheet' pinned to the wall.
- Comments can be invited as part of the introductions — 'My name is John, and I am here to learn . . .'

POINTS TO WATCH

☞ If done in a round, members tend to repeat what has been said before. Talking to a partner often elicits more accurate and interesting comments.
☞ At the beginning of a group, the stated reasons for attending are often rather limited. This may reflect a hazy idea of the benefit of pre-natal classes, or a lack of thought about personal goals.

SETTING AN AGENDA

AIMS

✓ To establish an agenda of topics to be discussed.
✓ To demonstrate negotiation in action.
✓ To encourage group participation, and a feeling of belonging within the group.

PROCESS

At the beginning of every class series, or perhaps at the start of every session within the series, the group negotiates a list of topics they want to discuss in the time available. If the list is long, it may be necessary to decide an order of priority or agree to omit some topics, which could be dealt with in other ways. This list may become the sole agenda for the session, or it could be used as an indicator for the topics which need special attention or which have special relevance for group members.

Use either a whiteboard or butcher's paper to record the suggested topics. When the full list is established, encourage discussion to develop priorities, negotiating (with respect to time available, equipment needed etc.) with the group if necessary.

VARIATIONS

- This activity can be presented as a small group discussion, useful if the group is very large. Smaller groups can report back and the suggestions can be summarised by the leader. These reports will often help in the prioritising process, since the number of identical responses will give an indication of their importance to the group.
- A possible list of topics can be prepared on paper, and circled or numbered by group members to indicate their priorities. The responses will need to be tallied by the leader and announced to the group, who may then need to negotiate the final agenda.

POINTS TO WATCH

- ☞ If you are using an agenda setting exercise, it is important to review the list at the end of the session to see if the group's needs have been met and to decide what to do about uncompleted agenda items.

GROUP RULES

AIMS

- ✓ To establish a framework for the group process.
- ✓ To identify ground rules for individual behaviour within the group setting.
- ✓ To provide a mechanism whereby the leader, or a group member, can intervene if necessary to maintain the group dynamics and process.

PROCESS

This activity works well if presented in conjunction with a group goal setting exercise.

Members are invited to identify acceptable behaviours for group participants. These are listed on butcher's paper and displayed prominently at all times during the group sessions.

Should it become necessary, the group rules can be invoked by the leader or any member of the group in order to bring unacceptable behaviours to the attention of everyone.

POINTS TO WATCH

☞ Make sure there is agreement before a group rule is recorded.

☞ Common group rules are: everyone has a right to be heard; taking turns; no 'put downs' of members; respect for individual opinions; 'right to pass'; keeping to time; sharing information; offering support. Other useful rules are: confidentiality (this can help promote a climate of trust); no smoking; wash up you own cup (or other housekeeping points).

GROUP GOALS

AIMS

✓ To establish some goals to be achieved as a group. These are different from personal goals, and focus more on social issues and group interactions.

✓ To introduce the concept of having goals, and the process of taking steps in order to achieve them.

PROCESS

This activity works well if presented immediately after the 'Group Rules' exercise.

Using butcher's paper to record the suggestions, invite the group members to think of outcomes they would like to achieve for the group. The list can be displayed alongside the Group Rules, as a reminder of one aspect of the group's focus.

POINTS TO WATCH

☞ Some people may be surprised that you have suggested that there may be goals for the group as well as for individuals. You may need to initiate some discussion centring around social support networks as a means of introducing the idea of goals for the group.

☞ Group goals might include: sharing of information; networking; increased confidence in teaching skills; mutual support; sharing of resources; having fun!

Identifying attitudes, values, feelings

People form a view about birth from a variety of inputs over many years. These often stem from experience, their cultural background, personal and family attitudes, specific information they have been given and personal expectations.

The results of these accumulated influences may have a profound effect on the way prospective parents approach parenthood and the birth experience. They may also colour their attitude to learning and to the group. It can be useful, therefore, to explore the views and feelings held by group members, to facilitate their participation and to help you provide appropriate information and support.

Choose these activities carefully. You may need to modify them to suit your particular group, and be alert to their reactions and their responses. Some of the following suggestions are best described as 'generic', since the activity can be adapted for a variety of topics. The process will be described here, followed by some suggestions for how these activities may be used in practice.

'What's on top?'

Aims

✓ To provide an opportunity for group members to state what is occupying their thoughts at a particular time, or an issue that is currently of concern.

✓ To foster feelings of openness in the group.

✓ To allow mutual sharing of problems and concerns.

Process

At the beginning of a session, members are invited to answer the question 'What's on top?' (In other words: 'What is uppermost in your mind at the moment?') Every member of the group is invited to participate and everything that is mentioned must be accepted, even if it is trivial or silly. The exercise may be completed as a round, with everyone taking a turn around the circle, or the invitation may be issued generally, with people invited to participate in any order. This approach may allow someone with a vital issue of concern to speak first.

POINTS TO WATCH

☛ Not everyone may wish to participate, and it should be acceptable to invoke the 'right to pass' rule (see exercise on Group Rules).

☛ If the leader begins, it will help break the ice, and establish the kind of information you are expecting from other group members (people tend to copy the kind of content offered by those who have spoken earlier).

☛ Try to avoid getting side-tracked onto discussion of issues that are raised. A comment such as 'Perhaps we should talk about that later' will help to keep the process going.

☛ Encourage people to open up by acknowledging their contribution — 'I can see that it has been a very difficult day for you', 'It sounds like that was quite an event!' etc.

TAKING A STAND

AIMS

✓ To offer an opportunity for individual group members to express an opinion.

✓ To enable the group to share views and explore attitudes, beliefs and values.

✓ To enable participants to hear other points of view on an issue and to expose people to different ideas.

✓ To provide a chance for everyone to participate, especially those who are often quiet or shy.

PROCESS

The leader has a set of five sheets of paper each describing a 'position':

- Agree
- Strongly agree
- Disagree
- Strongly disagree
- Don't know; not sure

These are arranged as stations on a circle, with enough space between to allow the group members to move around and stand in a chosen position.

The leader explains that the exercise is designed to explore views and opinions held by the group, and that a number of issues will be presented to the group for their consideration. Each member is then invited to 'take a stand' on the issue by choosing a position.

After everyone has found a position, the leader then invites each person to contribute their point of view (briefly). As each person speaks the leader makes no comment, except to thank the person for their statement.

When everyone has had their say, the leader introduces the next topic, waits for the group to reposition, and again invites comment. This continues until all the topics have been explored.

The leader then invites the group to comment on the activity and what they discovered. It may be decided to explore some issues further at a later time, particularly if specific information seems needed.

SUITABLE TOPICS

Choose issues or topics that will be familiar to the participants and on which they are likely to have an opinion. Avoid asking them to consider subjects are likely to be unfamiliar.

Suggestions: parenting issues (dummies, sleeping with the baby, leaving babies to cry, breastfeeding, spoiling etc.); birth (birth is a natural process, pain relieving drugs are OK, midwives are good at delivering babies, fathers should be at the birth, having an extra support person is helpful etc.).

VARIATIONS

If the group is large, to save time, all those standing on a particular position can discuss their reasons for their stance as a small group and present a summary to the large group.

POINTS TO WATCH

- ☛ The leader's role is to manage the process. Avoid being side-tracked into providing information — if the comments suggest that more information is needed or that myths need to be exposed, then schedule another time for this.
- ☛ Be very careful not to take sides. Be aware of your non-verbal messages as well as your spoken comments.
- ☛ If a verbal disagreement breaks out, especially between partners, use the group rules to restore order and to point out that everyone has the right to make their opinion known.
- ☛ If one person is left standing on a position on the opposite side to everyone else, quietly move beside them to lend physical support. You are not necessarily agreeing with them, but just offering your presence to reduce their discomfort from appearing at odds with the rest of the group.

☞ Group members may wish to invoke the 'Right to pass' group rule. People sometimes choose the 'Don't know' position to achieve the same end, and they should not be pressed to move elsewhere.

☞ Five or six issues are probably enough to explore in one session. Don't run the activity more than once in the class series.

'FIELD OF WORDS'

AIM

✓ To explore feelings generated by an activity or discussion topic.

PROCESS

Participants can be given a sheet of paper with a number of words scattered across the page. They are invited to consider a question and to circle those responses that apply to them. The prepared words should be related to feelings and contain equal numbers of positive and negative words (satisfied, contented, confused, overwhelmed, anxious, excited etc.). Possible topics could include 'How are you feeling now at the end of this session? 'How does this topic make you feel?'

Allow time to process the activity once it is completed, perhaps using a group discussion ('What did you find interesting about this activity?', 'What did you notice?' etc.) or even a sentence completion exercise (see below).

This activity can be also be adapted for use as an evaluation tool.

VALUES CLARIFICATION CARDS

AIMS

✓ To enable the group to explore attitudes and beliefs.
✓ To encourage small group discussion.
✓ To introduce the group to the process of coming to a consensus on an issue.

PROCESS

The leader prepares a set of cards, with each card in the set showing a word describing a feeling or emotion. The set has a balance of positive, negative and neutral words.

In small groups, the participants use the cards as the basis for a discussion on a given topic, and then arrange the cards in a visual representation of their collective viewpoint. This encourages small group interaction and requires negotiation to reach an acceptable group representation.

The words on the cards can be similar to those chosen for the 'field of words' exercise, and possible topics can include any of the suggestions listed in the 'Taking a stand' exercise or any other appropriate issue.

The group can also be given one or two additional blank cards so they can add words of their own choosing.

Each small group then displays their depiction to the larger group and explains the basis of their representation.

POINTS TO WATCH

☞ Choose topics that are likely to be familiar to the participants. As the leader, you must remain non-judgemental, and accept all comments neutrally.

☞ If you are providing a set of words to consider, make sure you provide a balance of positive, negative and neutral words. This will ensure that the group focuses on both sides of an issue, an important step in encouraging open, flexible attitudes.

☞ Finish the exercise by exploring the process involved in reaching agreement and discussing what was discovered through participation in the process.

SENTENCE COMPLETION

AIMS

✓ To provide a quick way to assess the current feelings in a group or to obtain quick feedback on an issue.

✓ To encourage individuals to contribute.

✓ To assess comfort levels, personal reactions and group responses to an activity.

PROCESS

Immediately following an activity on which you want feedback, provide members with pencil and paper and invite them to complete a sentence. Suitable sentence stems may include:

• 'Right now I am feeling . . .'
• 'I wish that I could . . .'
• 'Next session I hope that we . . .'
• 'The best thing about this topic was . . .'

- 'I was disappointed that . . .'
- 'Right now I want . . .'

Choose two or three sentence stems at the most, and try to balance a potential positive and negative response. When they have finished, participants can be invited to read their sentences aloud or, if preferred, can hand them in for the leader to read, either aloud or in private (this choice will depend on the purpose of the activity).

Points to watch

☛ Accept all responses neutrally, being aware of your non-verbal as well as verbal reactions.

☛ Participants may wish to exercise their 'right to pass', particularly if they have not been told in advance that they will be reading their sentence to the group. However, explaining in advance that sharing responses will be part of the exercise may encourage people to write sentences they consider 'acceptable', and this may defeat the aim of eliciting immediate, spontaneous reactions. You will have to decide which avenue to take, based on your objective for the exercise.

☛ Keep it light-hearted and accept all contributions, even those that say 'Right now I want to go home!'

☛ Remember that some people may have literacy problems with pencil and paper exercises.

Draw a picture

Aims

✓ To provide an alternative way of expressing feelings and emotions.

✓ To encourage participants to see 'the big picture' and to explore their place within it.

✓ To provide an activity that will interest the visually oriented style of learners.

Process

Participants are provided with large sheets of butcher's paper and crayons, pencils or pens in a variety of colours. They are invited to draw a picture on a specified topic or theme. They then explain their drawing to the rest of the group.

Possible topics: 'families', 'babies', 'our relationship', 'the way the pregnancy has changed our lives', 'becoming a parent', 'giving birth'.

VARIATIONS

- This can be done as a small group exercise, with a collective picture being assembled, following negotiation and discussion. Everyone should be encouraged to draw part of the picture.
- A collage could be assembled, using magazines and newspapers as a source of pictures and words.
- Participants could be invited to assemble 'found' objects to form a three dimensional representation — a 'still life' artwork.

POINTS TO WATCH

- ☛ Using a small group approach may help those who are shy about their artistic ability.
- ☛ Encourage abstract forms as well as realistic pictures, to take care of those who 'can't draw'.
- ☛ Allow plenty of time for the drawing or assembling as well as the explanation and sharing.

SMALL GROUP DISCUSSION

AIMS

- ✓ To encourage participation within the group.
- ✓ To explore topics of mutual interest, in a way in which everyone can contribute.
- ✓ To allow for individual expression within a very large group.
- ✓ To foster social support networks.
- ✓ To build trust in the group through sharing and listening.

PROCESS

The large group is divided into smaller groups comprised of either:

- Men and women in separate groups.
- Mixed small groups — with your partner.
- Mixed small groups — without your partner.
- Random groups. These can be made by numbering off around the big group, or by allocating people to groups according to 'favourite food' or 'holiday destination' etc., these designations having been offered by the group. For example: if five groups are needed, the leader asks for five favourite foods, then allocates everyone to a group of 'diners' using these nominated foods.

- Self selection. If small groups will be used several times, participants can be invited to make their own groups, 'choosing people whom you have not yet met', or 'choosing people with whom you haven't yet worked'.

The group is given a task, and a time limit. They are also asked to appoint a recorder who will report back the group's findings to the larger group when the time is up. The reports are read and discussed further if necessary, or if group consensus is desired.

POSSIBLE TOPICS

Almost any topic can be adapted for small group discussion. This process is particularly useful for involving everyone, especially if the main group is large. It is also a useful technique for sharing feelings and personal thoughts, especially when to reveal these in a large group may be inhibiting.

POINTS TO WATCH

☞ The groups must understand their task. The leader should explain the process and then, just after the activity has begun, check to make sure that each group understands what they have been asked to do.

☞ The leader should not participate in the small group discussion. It is important to allow the group to complete their task without the leader's input, to encourage free expression and to assist in the development of their own thoughts and ideas without the leader's influence.

☞ Small groups can be an inappropriate medium for problem solving, as there is a risk that misinformation and myths will be perpetuated. In addition, as a leader, you will have no idea what is being said, and will therefore be unable to correct facts or provide a more balanced viewpoint.

☞ When you are constructing your small groups, be aware that there will, in all likelihood, be different outcomes depending on the composition of the group. Separate sex groups often allow for more intimate discussion, and validate that men and women have different perspectives. When partners stay together in a small group it can be supportive, but also inhibiting if one partner is shy or domineering.

ACTIVITIES FOR INCREASING BODY AWARENESS AND PERSONAL INSIGHT

There are many ways to help women become more aware of their bodies and how they work during pregnancy and birth. Promoting insight into the physiology of having a baby may help increase confidence, an important pre-requisite for feeling empowered. All educators include physical exercises that involve women working with their bodies during pregnancy, and some of these, designed to meet specific objectives related to active birth, are described below. Other physical exercise programs can be found in the references listed at the end of this chapter.

AIMS

✓ To encourage participants to become aware of their own physical capabilities.

✓ To explore the effects of pregnancy on a woman's body.

✓ To encourage problem-solving through devising adaptations for physical limitations that may be present.

✓ To provide activities to boost confidence through the development of insight and an understanding of the anatomy and physiology of labour and birth.

✓ To encourage autonomy and the taking of responsibility during pregnancy, labour and birth.

✓ To encourage active participation in class, as part of the philosophy of active involvement in pregnancy, labour and birth.

✓ To allow partners to gain insights into the birth process, as a basis for providing support during labour.

SETTING THE SCENE FOR EXERCISE PROGRAMS

Involvement is an essential ingredient of exercise sessions. Everyone needs to participate, and gaining their co-operation is important, particularly at the beginning of the first exercise session, when people may still be shy.

Make sure that participants know there will be exercise sessions in advance and advise them to wear suitable clothes.

To encourage participation, introduce your activity carefully:

• Avoid giving the exercise a name or label, as this may raise concerns and anxieties.

- Have the group move to where they will be exercising (usually the floor), and begin by saying 'Let me show you something interesting . . .' or 'Let's have a look at this . . .'
- Check your own state: keep positive, encourage curiosity, make it serious, avoid being embarrassed, be open and enthusiastic.
- Try arranging the group members so they are looking at you, rather than each other (avoid exercising in a circle).

POINTS TO WATCH

☞ There will be moments when some participants may feel embarrassed. The simplest way to increase comfort is to ignore the resultant behaviour, and keep the exercise moving on. Drawing attention to possible feelings, making jokes, or singling out those who are embarrassed for attention, even by just making eye contact, can discourage participation.

☞ Try to avoid checking participants individually in a way that suggests you are assessing their performance. It is important to see that everyone is doing the exercise correctly but try to do this without creating an atmosphere of 'right' and 'wrong'.

☞ Be ready to assist those who are having trouble due to physical problems. Many people have stiff knees, ankles or hips and may find some exercises difficult. Others have bad backs. Instead of singling them out ('Would all those with back problems please wait until I can help you personally') encourage everyone to participate, and watch for those having difficulties. Help them to devise an adaptation to allow their continued participation — this is an important lesson for labour, when adaptation to the forces of contractions require a problem solving approach.

☞ Providing a hand-out will assist group members to remember the important points for completing an exercise correctly.

☞ Avoid telling group members what you want them to discover from doing an exercise. Encourage them to find the answers themselves — this is the basis of empowerment through the development of insight. Self directed learning is the most effective approach for adults. It will also avoid the potential of 'teacher knows best' or 'the teacher is the expert' that is inappropriate for adult learning.

TEACHING ANATOMY AND PHYSIOLOGY

Explaining the way a woman's body works during pregnancy, labour, birth and the post-partum period is a topic that will form one of the recurring themes of your classes.

AIMS

✓ To enable a woman to gain insight into the anatomy and physiology of pregnancy and birth.

✓ To empower her through knowledge.

✓ To assist her develop an appreciation of birth as a normal bodily process.

✓ To explore the variations that can occur during pregnancy and birth.

PROCESS

There are many ways in which you can explain anatomy and physiology. Since it can be a 'technical' topic, use visual aids to assist your presentation, and provide time for questions to clarify specific points or to provide additional information, as requested.

Since this is a large topic, break it into smaller subject areas and position it in the series when the information would be appropriate.

Creative use of teaching aids will be invaluable.

You could consider:

FETAL GROWTH AND DEVELOPMENT

* charts
* self examination
* photos of fetus
* models of growing baby

POSITIONS OF THE BABY AT TERM

* fetal doll and placenta against your own body
* fetal doll and pelvis
* diagrams or charts
* palpation of own tummy
* identification of fetal location and movement
* self examination of the cervix

THE STAGES OF LABOUR (OVERVIEW)

* knitted uterus and vagina

- chart showing time versus dilatation
- chart illustrating dilatation and effacement

BEHAVIOUR

- 'demonstrating' labour (see page 187)
- audiotapes of women in labour
- videotapes
- practising positions (see page 178), massage and self help ideas (see page 180)

MECHANICS OF SECOND STAGE

- self exploration of pelvic movement (see page 143)
- putting the fetal doll through the pelvis
- use of cloth perineal model to show crowning
- photographs
- video of birth
- chart showing cardinal movements

THIRD STAGE

- fetal doll and placenta, following from birth demonstration
- fetal doll put to breast

POINTS TO WATCH

☞ Be aware of your language: avoid jargon, emotionally laden comments and biassed remarks. You non-verbal communication also requires attention.

☞ Emphasise the positive aspects. Women need to feel inspired that their bodies can, and will, work well during labour.

☞ Be ready to deal with fears and worries expressed by group members. Many women, for example, are scared that their baby will not fit through the pelvis, and their feelings need to be acknowledged. Following up with a careful explanation of the anatomy involved and the development of a plan for helping themselves to avoid problems during labour may be helpful.

☞ Always begin with the normal anatomy and physiology before commenting on complications or variations. Try to keep a balanced perspective in the time allocated for these topics: if the birth process works well about 85–90% of the time, then this would be an appropriate proportion for the discussion time on this topic. Complications will therefore take up 10–15% of the available time, and not overpower the discussion with negative or unlikely eventualities.

LEARNING ABOUT THE PELVIS

This exercise demonstrates a number of important anatomical facts and enables women to discover how they can work with their bodies to get the baby through the pelvis. It is also useful for introducing concepts that will be explored in later sessions and to provide a framework for underpinning the main themes of active birth classes.

AIMS

✓ To show the anatomy of the pelvis and how the joints allow movement which can increase the internal space.

✓ To demonstrate that there are variations in individual pelvic shapes, and that external appearances have no bearing on internal capacities.

✓ To demonstrate the effects that various positions have on the pelvic bones and their ability to move.

✓ To help women get in touch with their bodies, and to have confidence in the way nature has designed the pelvis to assist in the birth process.

PROCESS

Have everyone on the floor, kneeling with their legs slightly apart. Include everyone in the class, not just the pregnant women. Using a pelvic model, tilt it to an angle of 45 degrees, as it is in the body, and indicate where the vertebrae continue from the top of the sacrum. Ask the group to use their own bodies to locate the landmarks as you show them on the model. Begin with the iliac crests from the anterior spine at the front. Using the thumbs, feel along the top of the crests around towards the back (figure 3).

Return to the anterior spine at the front and notice how the bone goes straight down at the front. Move your fingers down to locate the pubic bone. This is an important landmark as it locates the peak of the arch around which the baby pivots during second stage of labour (figure 4).

To locate the sacrum at the back of the pelvis, place your hand over the sacrum with the tips of the fingers in the crease between the buttocks. By moving the fingers down a little, it may be possible to feel the coccyx. Notice how your hand curves along the bone.

Leaving one hand on the sacrum, position the other hand on the pubic bone. With knees apart, bend forward slowly, then lean back. Observe the opening up of the space between the fingers when you bend forward and feel how the space closes up when you bend backwards (figure 5).

Have the group now sit on their heels with their knees together. Ask them to put their fingers into their buttocks to locate the ischial tuberosities (figure 6).

143

FIGURE 3

Locating the landmarks:

Begin with the iliac crests.

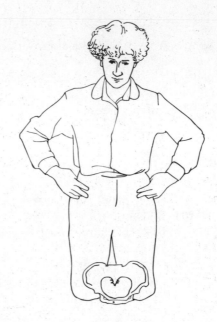

FIGURE 4

Move your fingers down to locate the pubic bone.

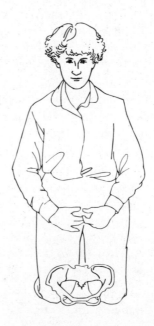

FIGURE 5

*With one
hand on the
pubic bone
and the other
over the
sacrum,
notice the
movement
when you
bend
forwards.*

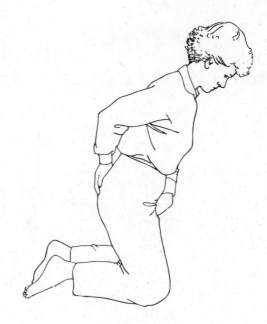

FIGURE 6

*Find the
ischial
tuberosities
while sitting
on your heels.*

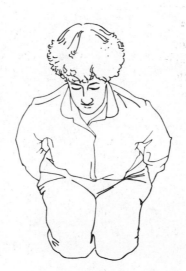

FIGURE 7

Explore the leverage on the pelvis created by moving your legs apart.

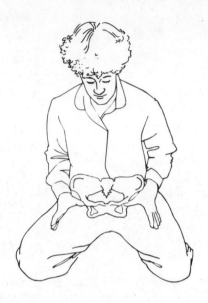

FIGURE 8

Semi-sitting puts all your body weight onto the sacrum and coccyx.

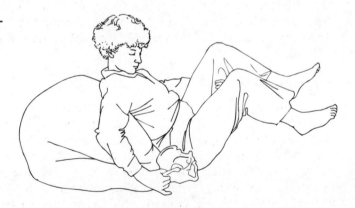

Leaving the fingers in place, and keeping the back straight, move the knees apart to a wide position while leaning slightly forward. Observe how the tuberosities swivel, and swing slightly apart. To explain why this happens demonstrate how this action is achieved through a leverage of the thigh bones against the sides of the pelvis at the hip joint (figure 7).

It is also assisted by the backwards motion of the sacrum when leaning forward. Show how sitting on the tuberosities makes this opening action more difficult due to the body weight which tends to impede the movement.

Ask the group to work out and show you which postures will allow the pelvis to open to its maximum capacity. Make sure they choose a pose which leaves the pelvis free to move, i.e. a position where they are weight-bearing on the legs. Have couples now experiment with different sitting positions. Observe that when completely upright, the sacrum and coccyx are free to move backwards because they are not weight-bearing. As the body is tilted backwards, the full weight is taken on the coccyx and sacrum and in order to balance (particularly if the feet are lifted off the floor) the abdominal and trunk muscles must be used (figure 8).

This semi-sitting position closes up the pelvis by forcing the sacrum and coccyx inwards. It feels uncomfortable and is an unstable position unless considerable effort is made to maintain balance. When lying flat with the knees bent it will be observed that again the coccyx and sacrum are free to move backwards as the body is now supported by the hip bones. With the legs lifted into a 'lithotomy' position, the pelvis is able to open fully. An emerging baby, however, would have to be propelled upwards against gravity during second stage and the weight of the baby against the inferior vena cava may reduce circulation to the placenta. In a side lying position the pelvis is also free to open up, especially if the top leg is lifted up and supported. The baby would need to be pushed along in a horizontal plane, without the assistance of gravity.

POINTS TO WATCH

☛ Some people in the group may be embarrassed by touching their bodies in this way. To help ease their discomfort and to give them non-verbal permission to participate, it's important for you to feel very comfortable handling your body, and to be unselfconscious during the demonstration. As you take the group through the exercise, maintain only general eye contact with the group. Sweep your gaze around without looking at any person in particular, and this will help you become aware of anyone who is feeling embarrassed. Don't make eye contact with someone who's feeling uncomfortable. This acknowledges their feelings, and may make them feel worse. Just allow them to participate at their own level.

☞ Try not to give the group answers or to predict what they will discover. Encourage them to form their own conclusions about the benefits of various positions and ask them to give you feedback about how their body feels when they are sitting on particular parts of their pelvis, imitating potential labour positions. The more you can encourage the couples to think these points through, the greater will be the impact of your message.

☞ The men in the group need to understand the advantages of an upright posture so that they will feel confident in supporting their partner in her chosen position for labour and birth when the time comes. You can increase his interest in the exercise by including words and phrases designed to catch his attention, such as 'mechanics (of the birth process)', 'leverage (caused by the thigh bones)', 'construction (of the pelvis)', 'design (of the bony shapes)' etc.

☞ For the woman, seeing the potential of her body movements will encourage her to remain upright and active during labour and birth, and also to improve her body's abilities further through stretching exercises in pregnancy. Choose your descriptive words to enhance the potential of her body, and avoid negative phrases. For example, when describing the purpose of the curve of the sacrum, explain that it 'directs the baby's movements' and that the baby will 'slide down the inside of the bone and be directed forwards towards the exit'. Using the word 'slide' instead of 'push' sounds much less difficult, whilst still being anatomically correct. In pointing out the bony protuberances (ischial spines) tell her that this is 'the narrowest point the baby will need to negotiate', rather than indicating that is the place where some babies get stuck. Try to include words such as 'roomy', 'clever design', 'flexible capacity' and 'potential' in your accompanying description during the exercise.

☞ At the end of the exercise, invite discussion about what has been noticed or discovered by group members. You may be asked to explain why women are often asked to lie down for second stage when it is clearly more advantageous to be upright for birth. If you are asked this question, try reflecting it back to the group for consideration, rather than providing an answer yourself. A lively discussion may result, during which the politics of birth may be raised. Exploring this aspect of birth can provide valuable insights, important for the empowerment process.

PREGNANCY EXERCISE

Most pre-natal classes include a component on pregnancy exercise. Since the time available is often limited, educators have to make a decision about what to include. Special exercise classes (yoga, aquarobics etc.) may be available in the community for those who want more time for exercises than can be provided in the pre-natal setting.

Since participating in exercise offers an ideal way for women to become more aware of their pregnant bodies, and there are important benefits to be gained from exercise during pregnancy, the following activities should be considered for inclusion in your program.

STRETCHING EXERCISES

The exercises explained in this manual form the basis of a simple stretching program for pregnancy. There are many other possible exercises that could be included and resources for exercise in pregnancy are listed at the end of this chapter.

AIMS

✓ To increase awareness of the flexibility provided by the pregnancy hormones.
✓ To provide exercises that can ease some of the side effects of pregnancy.
✓ To encourage an understanding of the body's capacities.

PROCESS

The exercises described below are divided into two general sections. The first group are intended for the woman to work at on her own; for the exercises in the second group she will need to have a partner.

Invite everyone in the class to participate. The men will better understand the purpose of the exercise and everyone will get the benefits of stretching, which is useful for the release of any muscular tension. The women will find they stretch more easily because they are pregnant, and this can build confidence and boost morale.

TAILOR SITTING

This exercise involves sitting with the soles of the feet together with your heels as close to your body as can be comfortably achieved. It's important that your back be straight. To help adopt the right position of feet and back, put your hands beside your bottom, on the floor. This will not only keep your

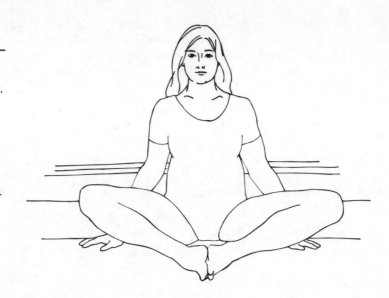

FIGURE 9

Tailor sitting.

Back straight, feet together, against a wall or unsupported.

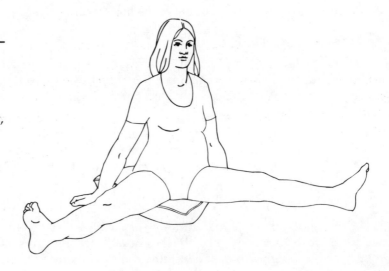

FIGURE 10

Sitting with legs apart.

Back straight, slide forward off pillow for extra stretch.

FIGURE 11

Japanese sitting:

begin by sitting on your heels.

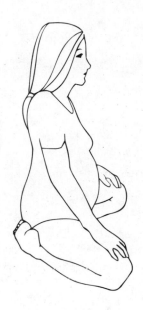

FIGURE 12

Slide hands forward, keeping your bottom on your heels.

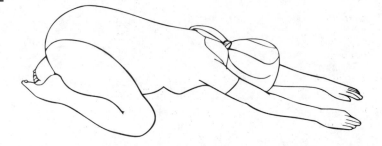

FIGURE 13

*Bend elbows
to rest in this
position.*

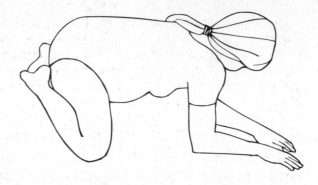

FIGURE 14

*Follow on to
pelvic
rocking,
moving knees
together
until under
your hips.*

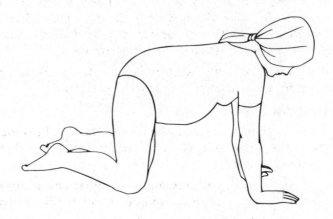

FIGURE 15

*Round your
back then
return to
level.*

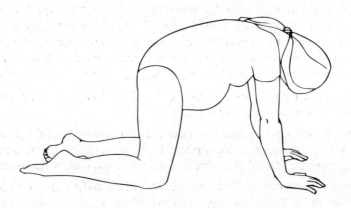

back straight, but by lifting your bottom, it can be moved closer to your feet, which will help with the initial positioning (figure 9).

It is very important to refrain from bouncing the knees. There seems to be a natural tendency to want to bounce, but this causes potential strain on the muscles of the inner thigh, and can cause over-stretching and joint damage. When the knees are bounced, the muscles are stretched in a way similar to the action of pulling on a rubber band. When bouncing the tension is maintained in the muscles to protect them from being over-stretched, and this counteracts the aim of the exercise, which is to allow the legs to just fall open with the weight of the knees stretching the muscle to its maximum length.

SITTING WITH LEGS APART

A pillow will be necessary for this exercise. Sit on the corner of the pillow with the legs as wide apart as possible and toes pointing upwards. Put your hands on the floor at the side. Hold that position for about 10 or 20 seconds, and then, using your hands to lift your bottom off the pillow, slide it forward onto the floor itself. An extra stretch will result (figure 10).

Hold this position, and observe how, after about 20 seconds, the pain starts to ease as the muscle relaxes in its newly stretched state.

JAPANESE SITTING

Japanese sitting begins a series of exercises that can be done in progression. Begin by sitting on your heels, with toes pointing together and the knees spread wide apart (figure 11).

If that is a comfortable position, and is easily achieved, try moving the feet slightly apart so that you can sit your bottom on the floor between them.

Some people will have difficulty with this exercise, particularly those who have stiff knees or large leg muscles. They can be helped by putting a rolled up pillow underneath their bottom to sit on, or by placing a pillow behind each knee. This will ease the pressure on the knee joints, and will help them to gradually become accustomed to the extra stretch. Manually rolling the calf muscle out to each side before settling back on to the heels may also help.

Slide your hands forward along the floor, keeping your back straight and your bottom on your heels (figure 12).

Go as far as you can, until you can rest your elbows on the floor for additional support. Keeping the chin up and looking forward will help to remind you to keep your back straight, which is an important part of this exercise (figure 13).

Rest in that position for a few minutes, then swing up onto hands and knees. At this point it may be necessary to bring the knees closer together, under the hip joints (figure 14).

Once on hands and knees, the exercise progresses into a series of pelvic rocking movements. Begin by rounding the back, and tucking the head and bottom under. Return to the level position (figure 15).

Watch the group as they do this exercise, and check that no-one is allowing their back to sag towards the floor. This will cause over-stretching of ligaments in the spine and can add to backache problems rather than relieve them. Once the general action of this exercise has been established, do it rapidly a number of times and the class couples will feel a pelvic rocking action.

Next try 'wagging' your tail. Turn your head to look at your right hip as you swing it towards your head, then turn your head to the other side as you swing your left hip towards your head. Again, once the basic action has been understood, do it quickly a number of times and you will feel that sensation of your tail wagging, as the muscles on each side of your spine receive a useful lateral stretch.

The last exercise that can be shown on hands and knees is to make circles with your bottom, in a gentle, belly dance action. Move in both directions, and feel the pelvis being mobilised in all directions. At the conclusion of the exercise, sit back on your heels.

You may find people in the group who have difficulty doing this exercise due to knee injuries, or back problems. As with all these exercises, don't discourage them from attempting it initially. Many women need to find ways of labouring on hands and knees or kneeling, therefore it is important that people who do have physical problems find ways of adapting these positions to take maximum advantage of gravity and mobility during their labour. You may need to assist them with this, using pillows under their knees, additional support from beanbags, or modifying the exercise slightly so that they can work at their maximum potential.

It is worthwhile pointing out that this hands and knees activity is good not only for relieving backache: it will also help general stiffness that occurs in the spine and neck as a result of chronic low backache, and it will also help the baby to turn into a favourable anterior position. You can demonstrate this using a fetal doll against your own body as you bend forward onto hands and knees.

As part of the discussion surrounding this exercise, it can be useful to explain the increased curvature in the spine that occurs as a result of the weight of the growing baby pulling forward on the spine, and the compensating action of throwing the shoulders back to maintain balance. You may also like to remind the group that the ligaments that support the uterus are attached to each side of the sacrum, and that as the baby grows, there will be extra strain on these ligaments, and on the sacral area. All the ligaments and muscles supporting the spine and pelvis are softened by the pregnancy hormones, and whilst this is essential for extra flexibility and mobility in labour, it does mean that some women suffer from extra backache and increased discomfort at the pubic joint and in their lower back during pregnancy.

BACK EXERCISES

These two exercises are designed to relieve backache, increase muscle strength and improve mobility.

The first one begins with lying on your back, knees up, and hands at your side. Pull your buttocks together tightly, and then lift your hips and roll your weight up your spine until you are supporting your body on your feet and upper back. The baby will tend to tip up off the pubic joint, which will relieve some pressure in that area. Hold the position for a few minutes, and then roll back down, releasing the buttocks last (figure 16).

The second exercise is done with your legs crossed and your feet hooked together at the ankles. By making small circles with the feet, as though you were drawing circles on the floor with a pencil gripped between your ankles, it is possible to give your lower back a massage. Keep your knees forward over your chest to take the weight of your legs off your abdominal muscles. The best massage in this position will be obtained if you lie on a firm surface, not on a soft mattress (figure 17).

Before beginning both of these exercises, show the women how to roll onto their backs from a side sitting position and remind them to roll over to the side before sitting up at the completion of the exercise. It is important not to sit straight up from a recumbent position as this places excessive strain on the abdominal muscles, and has the potential to cause damage.

STRETCHING AGAINST THE WALL

This is a very popular exercise with most pregnant women, because it is very good for relieving tired legs, for helping circulation, and for giving a measure of relief to varicose veins, both of the legs and in the vulva. You will need a suitable wall area to demonstrate this exercise and for the group to use during practice.

Begin by demonstrating the starting position: sit sideways against the wall, raising the hip against the wall up off the floor. Put one hand in front and the other hand behind to support yourself, and then as you turn and lift your legs, swing your body round, and your buttocks should finish up against the wall in the right position. Practise this a few times. If you end up with your buttocks a few centimetres from the wall, try again, making sure that the hip against the wall is lifted up high enough before you start (figure 18).

FIGURE 16

Back exercises.

Lifting buttocks off the floor.

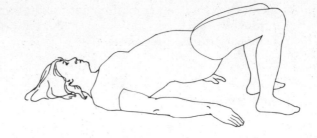

FIGURE 17

Massage your lower back by making circles with your feet.

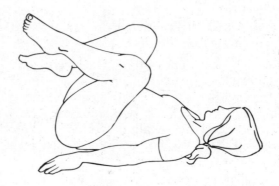

FIGURE 18

Stretching against the wall.

Begin like this, with your legs straight.

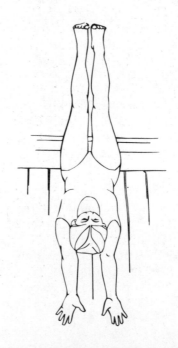

FIGURE 19

This is the stretching position.

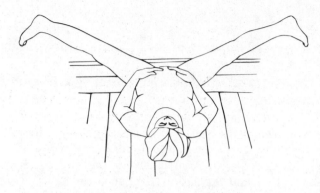

FIGURE 20

A resting position.

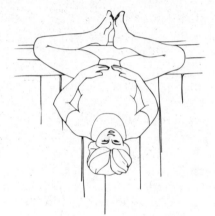

FIGURE 21

Resting as though 'sitting' against the wall.

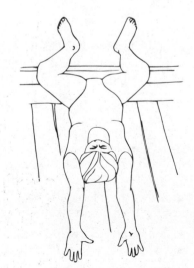

Straighten your legs, and then allow them to flop open into the stretching position (figure 19).

There are two possible resting positions: either 'sitting' against the wall, or with your legs in a tailor sitting position (figures 20 & 21).

When the hands are extended above the head, it is possible for a partner to apply a little spinal traction by pulling on your wrists sufficiently to just slightly move your buttocks away from the wall. Have the partner release your wrists, and enjoy the feeling of your spine being fully extended and supported on the floor. Most women find this extremely comfortable, as it relieves backache, provides pelvic tilt which helps to relieve feelings of pressure in the lower pelvic region, and circulation is enhanced by having your legs elevated. A woman who has problems with swelling in her ankles and who is told to put her feet up could try this exercise, which may be more effective in relieving the problem than lying on a bed or sitting in a chair with her feet on a footstool.

Occasionally, a woman might discover that lying on her back in this way causes dizziness when she rolls over to the side and sits up, especially in late pregnancy. This is because the weight of the baby presses on the major blood vessels returning through her body to the heart. This problem may be relieved by placing a firm pillow or a rolled up towel underneath the left buttock. The body will be on a slight sideways tilt, and by shifting the baby slightly to the right side, the pressure will be taken off the blood vessels which run up the left side of the body towards the heart. However, any woman who still has a problem or finds this exercise uncomfortable should use her common sense and refrain from practising it.

TWISTING

This exercise gives a good lateral stretch to the muscles that run up either side of the spine. Starting from a supine position (remember to demonstrate the correct way to get up and down) with the knees bent and the feet as close as possible to your bottom, swing your knees first to one side and then the other. As the knees drop to the floor, keep your feet together — the top foot will lift off the floor. Keep your shoulders on the floor at all times.

The weight of the knees may be enough to stretch the muscles in the lower back, and some people also feel a stretch towards the shoulder blades. If there is little stretch, use the hand on the same side as the knees to pull the knees up, along the floor, towards the hand. Keep the other arm on the floor to maintain both shoulders against the floor (figure 22).

A partner can increase the stretch by applying a little pressure against the knees and the opposite shoulder, on the floor (figure 23).

FIGURE 22

Dropping your knees to the side will give a lateral stretch to your back.

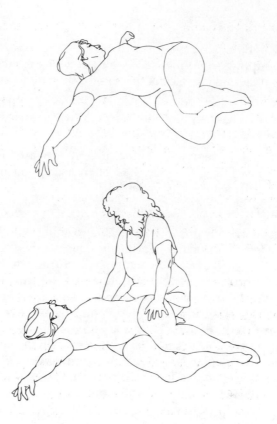

FIGURE 23

A partner can increase the stretch like this.

FIGURE 24

Loosen up your calf muscles before squatting.

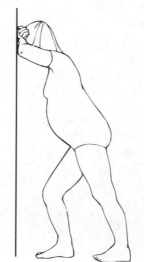

Calf stretches

For many people, squatting may be difficult, and as a warm up measure before attempting squatting, some calf stretching exercises will help to prepare the muscles up the back of the legs for the extended stretch they will feel when squatting.

These calf stretches can be done in several ways, and the simplest way is to stretch supported by the wall (figure 24).

Make sure that the feet are pointing directly forward, and that the weight is taken on the back leg. If no stretch is felt, it usually means that the toes of the back foot are turned slightly to the side.

Squatting

Some people in your group will be able to squat with ease and others may have considerable difficulty in achieving this position. Explain to the women that since they will always be supported during squatting in labour, even women who normally have difficulty assuming this position will find it is possible during birth, should they find this position helpful. The reason for practising squatting in pregnancy is mainly to develop flexibility in the ankles, knees and calf muscles and to become familiar with the position. It is unnecessary to be able to squat unsupported with the heels flat on the floor as the essential element is being able to adopt a position where the knees are higher than the hip joints. This will enable the greatest leverage, and therefore opening, of the pelvic bones during labour.

There is a difference between squatting with the heels up and with the heels down. When the heels are lifted off the floor, it is necessary to use muscle power to maintain balance. It is quite an active position and allows easy movement of the body and swivelling of the hips, and so on. With the heels down, the muscles stretch and relax, and this is a resting position. By clasping the hands at the front, using your elbows on the inside of your knees, and leaning forward, squatting with the heels down may be easier to maintain. For those people in the group who are having difficulty squatting unsupported, demonstrate how to use a chair, the wall, a low footstool or telephone book to take their weight. Alternatively, try resting the heels on a book or rolled up towel (figure 25).

Since a pregnant woman's circulation tends to be a little sluggish due to the pregnancy hormones, remind women to avoid squatting for more than a few minutes at a time. This will reduce the risk of varicose veins developing and avoid deep pelvic congestion.

FIGURE 25

There are many ways to achieve a squatting 'shape', either on your own or using furniture, a book or chair, for support.

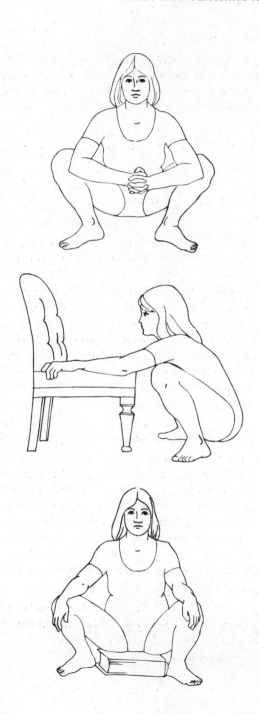

POINTS TO WATCH

☞ Some people find participating in exercise programs embarrassing. Invite the group to join in, but don't insist if someone wishes to sit this part of the class out. A private discussion at an appropriate time may reveal the reason for their unwillingness to join in. Not being able to participate can also be a source of embarrassment, and you should be sensitive to this possibility, perhaps suggesting adaptations of the exercises or providing a means of increasing their comfort that will make participation possible, particularly if their reluctance to join the group stems from a physical problem.

☞ Wearing suitable clothing, having enough space and facing away from the group when sitting with legs open, for example, will also make participation more comfortable.

☞ You will need plenty of space for some exercises. If floor or wall space is limited, it may be better to omit some exercises rather than ask your group to perform them in cramped conditions. Sufficient space for your exercise program will be one of your considerations in choosing a suitable venue.

☞ Make sure that everyone understands each exercise and how to perform it correctly. This is especially important for practising at home, unsupervised. After you have demonstrated each exercise, explaining the important points, watch the group as they try them out, checking that they have understood your instructions. Gently and unobtrusively correct those who need it, avoiding singling them out in the group.

☞ The onus on whether these exercises are practised at home should rest with your clients. Taking care of themselves during pregnancy is part of assuming responsibility for their own comfort and has implications for labour as well. There is no need for you to quiz your group on whether they have been practising at home — this kind of approach can be an unwelcome reminder of school homework!

☞ These are the most basic stretching exercises that can be taught in prenatal classes. Encourage your couples to practice them by combining their exercise session with some other activity, such as watching television, talking on the telephone, reading books to small children, etc. Most people don't have time in their busy days to schedule a specific 15 or 20 minute exercise program, but most people do spend at least some time each day watching the news or a favourite program on television, and by using the commercial breaks or changes in news story as a signal to change position or go on to the next exercise, it is very easy to go through all of these exercises in the space of one short viewing session.

☞ In addition to showing your class these exercises, it is worthwhile mentioning the importance of posture: keeping the back straight with chin tucked in, tucking the buttocks under and thinking 'tall'. Wearing low heeled shoes will avoid excessive forward tilting of the hips and strain on the legs.

☞ In *Preparing for Birth* there are some extended stretches illustrated at the end of the general stretching section. These extended stretches can be used not only to increase the amount of flexibility and mobility in the pregnant woman's body, but also as a practice session for coping with pain in labour. The use of these extended stretching exercises will be explained in a later section of this manual that deals with teaching about pain in labour.

GENERAL EXERCISE IN PREGNANCY

Apart from doing stretching exercises each day pregnant women may find it helpful to incorporate some general exercise into their daily routine. This can improve general circulation, relieve fatigue, and help the baby into a good position, especially towards the end of pregnancy.

Suggesting a general exercise program must not, however, link physical fitness with a better birth outcome: there is no evidence that being physically fit improves endurance during labour or makes the birth faster or easier. Every baby will be born when the time is right, regardless of whether the mother is fit or not, and general exercise is more useful for relieving the minor discomforts of pregnancy that occur day to day. Using the analogy of a fitness program in pregnancy as being similar to preparing for a 'marathon' race may engender fear and guilt in those who are disinclined to exercise, and in any case the pregnancy hormones appear to encourage sedate and less physically risky behaviours in pregnant women. As the muscles and ligaments soften towards the end of pregnancy, the joints are less well supported and are more vulnerable to injury from inappropriate exercise. The changes in the metabolism that occur naturally in pregnancy simulate mild aerobic exercise, and increasing this load may be uncomfortable or unwise for some women. Anyone with doubts about their fitness should consult a doctor or a physiotherapist who can advise on appropriate levels of exercise and prescribe suitable programs.

Some women will have been working through a general exercise program before pregnancy, perhaps including jogging or aerobics, yoga, etc. There is no reason why these forms of activity cannot be continued through the pregnancy provided the mother is healthy and the instructor is made aware of the pregnancy. Some specific exercises, particularly in aerobics and yoga, will be unsuitable due to the extra stretchiness of the ligaments as a result of the pregnancy hormones. As pregnancy advances a woman will find that her endurance level drops, so she needs to be prepared to alter her activity level according to her capacity. This tuning in to her body during the pregnancy is a way of preparing her for a similar approach during labour.

For those women who have not been exercising regularly this time of pregnancy can be used to develop a regular exercise routine. A woman's attention is centred on her body during this time, and therefore she may be more open to suggestions about exercising, particularly if it will help alleviate some of the discomforts of pregnancy. After the baby is born it is useful for mothers to continue with daily exercise, not only as a way of getting out and meeting people, but also to counter fatigue that is common in the first few months after the baby arrives.

The most suitable exercises for pregnant women, especially those who have not already been involved in an exercise program, are walking and swimming. Both of these activities involve large muscle groups in the body and provide general stimulation to circulation as well as gently increasing the heart rate and lung capacity. Walking involves a brisk walk of a couple of kilometres, not a gentle leisurely stroll. It is important to wear flat-heeled shoes when walking, and to move along at a comfortable pace.

Swimming is ideal for pregnant women because the buoyancy provided by the water allows a freedom of movement that is unattainable on land, and provides relief from the weight of the baby. Any swimming stroke is suitable, and a woman should just work at her own pace in the water, swimming laps or doing some general stretching and exercising in the water. If the membranes have ruptured or if there is a hind waters leak, then swimming is to be avoided, but otherwise it can be continued right through the pregnancy, even in the early part of the first stage of labour. It would be helpful to have a list of local heated swimming pools available, so that women know where they can swim in the winter months. Some pools even have special 'aquarobics' groups designed especially for pregnant women.

PELVIC FLOOR EXERCISES

The pelvic floor is automatically exercised when a woman walks, swims or does aerobics, yoga, etc. In fact, this is probably the most convenient way in which to exercise the pelvic floor.

AIMS

✓ To explain the role and function of the muscular basin that supports the abdominal organs during childbirth.

✓ To enable women to learn how to regain good muscle tone in this area after the baby is born, as a means of avoiding problems with incontinence and to reduce the potential for prolapse of the uterus in later life.

✓ To increase circulation in the pelvic region, helpful in promoting the healing following an episiotomy or repair of a tear, by reducing bruising.

PROCESS

Sit on a hard chair with your legs spread wide and your elbows resting on your knees. Your pelvic floor muscles should be resting against the seat of the chair.

Imagine that you are trying to prevent diarrhoea, or the passing of wind.

Tighten the muscles around the anus, and also the front passage (as though you are trying not to wet your pants in an emergency). As you tighten, lift all the muscles in the area up off the chair. Hold while you count slowly towards 10 (you may only make it as far as 4, 6 or 8, depending on the strength of these muscles). Release and rest for 4 seconds.

Repeat, contracting and lifting the muscles until they fatigue. Aim to reach a set of 6 contractions in succession.

Repeat this set several times a day, with an overall goal of holding each contraction for up to 10 seconds, with 6–8 contractions in each set. If the muscles are weak at the beginning, it may take several weeks to reach this goal.

POINTS TO WATCH

☛ In the post-partum period the simplest way for a mother to exercise her pelvic floor muscles is to go for a brisk walk each day with the baby in a pram. If there is felt to be any weakness in the pelvic floor muscles, however, or any symptoms of incontinence, then specific pelvic floor exercises are essential for rehabilitation of these muscles. Women who suffer from stress incontinence during the pregnancy, often made worse by the increasing weight of the baby pressing against the bladder, should also find this exercise beneficial.

☛ Many women have weak pelvic floor muscles, often causing acute embarrassment and discomfort from stress incontinence. You can assist by providing a list of incontinence advisers, physiotherapists who specialise in this area of women's health, or doctors with a special interest in bladder problems, and encouraging these women to seek help.

Perineal massage

Although doing perineal massage for the last weeks of pregnancy will not guarantee that a tear can be avoided, massaging encourages couples to take responsibility for birth preparation, accustoms the woman to the sensations that she will feel in second stage, and thus will help to allay fears of pain at this time in labour.

Aims

✓ To encourage body awareness in pregnant women.

✓ To increase stretchiness of the vaginal opening, which may reduce the likelihood of perineal trauma during birth.

✓ To familiarise women with the sensations caused by extended stretching of the perineum, as a means of reducing fear during second stage.

Process

This topic can be introduced into pre-natal classes towards the end of the series, particularly when explaining ways to avoid episiotomy and other perineal trauma in second stage. Because perineal massage doesn't need to be done for more than the last four or five weeks of the pregnancy, you can leave mentioning it until the last weeks of your classes when your couples will probably be at the right stage of the pregnancy to begin doing this simple exercise.

Since you will not actually be demonstrating the exercise to the group you will need a diagram or a knitted uterus with the vaginal extension to show what is meant by perineal massage. Explain that the massage is done by the woman herself using a suitable oil, preferably of vegetable origin, as a lubricant. Using her thumbs, she gently stretches the perineum to the point where the skin feels tense with a hot, burning feeling. Massage for a few minutes at this point of maximum stretch to become accustomed to the sensations. Having a diagram to follow and some written instructions is very helpful, and these can be found in *Preparing for Birth*.

Points to watch

☞ Some women find the whole idea of touching their bodies in this way quite distasteful. Try to avoid colourful language, introduce the idea gently, and suggest that it is an exercise to try privately, at home.

TEACHING ABOUT PAIN

For first time parents-to-be the pain of labour is an unknown quantity, something to be wondered at, or even feared. Since pain is often seen as negative and unproductive, many women are extremely anxious about managing their reactions to labour.

In choosing group activities, therefore, it is important not to feed into this negativism and to avoid activities that invite people to imagine catastrophes. Even drawing on past experience as a basis for predicting responses in labour has its problems — labour pain has a different quality to other pain and stems from a different physiological basis. It is impossible to predict how much labour will hurt, or how the contractions will be registered by an individual. Therefore an emphasis on activities that are anchored in concepts, and are designed to explore attitudes, encourage participants to build a repertoire of self-help measures that can be adapted as needed, encourage an open mind about eventual labour patterns and focus on the positive, problem-solving aspects of management, may offer more benefit to parents.

In focusing on the pain of labour the aim is to:

✓ Explore attitudes and beliefs about pain in labour.

✓ Devise self-help strategies that may be used to manage labour pain.

✓ Explore concepts about pain management — relaxation, being open minded, trusting that the body is working normally.

✓ Provide information about the physiological basis for pain in labour.

✓ Correct misinformation, and provide positive inputs about the nature and purpose of pain in labour.

There are a number of ways these aims can be achieved.

LECTURETTE

As a preface to any activities that explore pain management in detail, a short lecturette on the physiology of pain may be useful. Few people have considered the purpose of pain in labour, and their fears may be based on distorted beliefs and misinformation.

AIMS

✓ To describe the physiology of labour pain: why it is part of the birth process; what triggers the painful feelings; the role of endorphins; the effects of adrenalin on pain perception.

✓ To dispel myths and provide a factual basis for exploration of self-help measures.

PROCESS

A lecturette is a short lecture, perhaps lasting no more than 15 minutes. Provide a simple outline of the basic facts and allow time for questions to expand the topic.

POINTS TO WATCH

☞ You should pay particular attention to the language you use and your non-verbal communications. Note the reactions of the group and of the individuals to your words.

☞ Pay attention to any feelings being expressed, and be alert for questions that reflect cultural practices that may be relevant when discussing self-help measures later.

☞ Look for later opportunities to reinforce your message or remind the group of the factual basis of pain, particularly when practising positions, or discussing aids to relaxation, the role of support people and obstetric interventions and drugs.

DISCUSSION

Discussion on pain may be best managed in the large group, to avoid the risk of reinforcement of misinformation and myths that could happen in small, unsupervised groups.

AIMS

✓ To encourage participants to explore attitudes to pain, and the basis of beliefs about pain in labour.

✓ To provide an opportunity for participants to hear other people's views, as a means of broadening their experience.

✓ To encourage the exploration of fears and anxieties about managing labour pain.

PROCESS

You will need to provide an activity to start the discussion: a short video showing women in first stage; a brainstorm on the word 'labour' or 'contractions', a story about one woman's labour (perhaps a labour report, or an excerpt from a novel), etc.

Invite participation using an appropriate general question, for example: 'How does it feel to watch someone in labour as we saw on the video?', 'How could we summarise these words you have presented on pain?', 'How does this story about labour make you feel?'. Allow enough time for everyone to have their say. When you are ready to close the activity, you will need to summarise the discussion before moving the group on to the next topic.

POINTS TO WATCH

☞ Be prepared to use silence. If the group is reluctant to start, just wait. Someone will eventually begin! Be aware of your own non-verbal behaviour while you wait — if you start looking anxious or impatient, you will inhibit participation. Sometimes the silence just reflects the need to think, or that people need time to formulate a response.

☞ Try to encourage everyone to have a say. If one or two dominate the discussion, gently invite others to participate, perhaps by using their names to catch their attention.

☞ If necessary, use the Group Rules (see above) to encourage everyone to join in and to limit domination by a few.

USING EXTENDED STRETCHES

Finding a suitable way of simulating contractions and illustrating the importance of relaxation as a tool for coping with pain has always been a difficult task for childbirth educators. In the past, many chose 'Chinese burns', thigh pinching, holding ice cubes, or something similar, as a means of simulating labour contractions. These methods have one major problem, however. They do not provide a realistic simulation of contractions and because they seem somewhat irrelevant, couples do not always take this activity seriously, or make the connection between thigh pinching, for example, and labour contractions.

Using extended stretches offers a more realistic approach: during the exercise muscles are being stretched in an area adjacent to the cervix, and this provides a sensation similar to the pain emanating from the stretching cervix during labour.

AIMS

✓ To encourage the group to explore the physical sensations caused by stretching muscle.

✓ To focus attention on the concept of accepting the pain, not fighting it.

✓ To explore the role of relaxation (mental) as a management tool for labour.

✓ To analyse the role of support people during labour.

PROCESS

Ask couples to sit opposite their partner facing each other as illustrated. Have the men experience the stretch first, because their lack of suppleness often makes this exercise more difficult for them, and, having experienced the stretch themselves, they will be better placed to understand the need for gentleness with their pregnant partners when it is their turn (figure 26).

Position the man as shown above, with the legs wide apart and his partner's feet against his calves. She should grip him round the wrists so that his hands are relaxed and she is supporting the full weight of his arms and shoulders.

Begin by doing some warm-ups — have the partner swing him around in circles, gently stretching the inner thigh muscles. Make circles in both directions.

Next, have the partner slowly lean back, pulling on his wrists, to bring him forward. Ask the men to indicate when the point of maximum stretch is reached. Hold at that point for about 10 seconds. Both partners should now become aware of the stretch — how it feels, and how far forward he has moved.

Take a short break and explain that next time when he feels that stretch coming, you will offer some ideas for helping him to manage the stretch. Have the partner begin to exert the stretch, and as she does so, ask the man to close his eyes, allow his shoulders to drop, and feel his body getting softer, limper, and heavier with each breath out. Use the breath to release the tension. As the stretch is maintained, continue to talk him through, encouraging him to feel his body opening and becoming relaxed and floppy. Let the stretch continue for about a minute (although do not necessarily time this) and then ask the group to take a rest.

FIGURE 26

Extended stretch exercise.

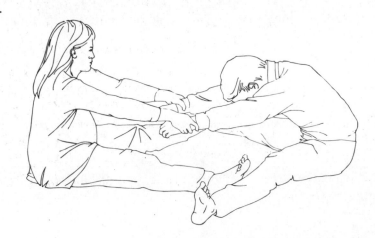

At this point, ask the group if they noticed any differences when doing the exercise the second time. Allow everybody to discuss this with their partner and to share their findings with the group. Many will say that they found that they could stretch a little further. Some may report that although the pain was still there, they felt it was not as intense the second time. The women may report that they could feel their partner 'giving' with each out breath and that they could see his head flopping further forward towards the floor.

Ask the group to ready themselves for one final stretch. Again, as you take them through this third stretch, talk them through, using words such as 'open', and 'giving', 'feeling heavy', 'loose', 'limp', 'feeling their body', 'working well', 'going with it', 'not fighting it', 'letting the stretch happen', and 'becoming flexible and soft'. Avoid using the word 'relaxation', which is not particularly descriptive for many people. As the stretch reaches a maximum, encourage the men to make a noise in their throat, either a sighing, grunting or moaning sound. Partners can be invited to accompany them. Allow the stretch to continue a little longer than the earlier stretch, and encourage the couples to 'stay with it — it's an extra strong stretch and it's still there — allow it to happen — feel your body working through it — it feels good — it's working well'. At the end of the stretch, allow everybody time to share their feelings with each other, and then to share them with the group. Many couples will report that they were able to achieve an extra stretch once they made some noise.

Other 'discoveries' couples may make include:

- it is difficult to make noise in public (yet this is what will need to happen during labour),
- making noise helps to increase the relaxation (sportsmen do this under extreme physical strain),
- it is important to feel that your partner is with you, not only physically, but mentally (many couples are helped if you encourage the partner to breathe along or make an accompanying noise as the exercise progresses),
- you can achieve more with a stronger stretch at the end of the exercise than you could at the beginning (this has analogies with labour — when the first few contractions have been felt, and a woman finally knows what she will be working with, can she really let herself go).

The rate of breathing is unimportant. The aim of this exercise is to visualise the out breath as a way to release tension. Sometimes couples will notice that as the stretch becomes stronger, the rate of breathing increases slightly. This is a normal response in the body and will happen automatically during labour. This approach is completely opposite to the patterned breathing used in psychoprophylaxis, when the emphasis on short, staccato breaths, accentuating the in breath as much as the out breath, resulting in a state of inner tension rather than relaxation.

This exercise also simulates labour from the earlier, simple contractions through to the more difficult and lengthy transition contractions. By getting used to stretch in this progressive way couples find they can achieve more progressively by just going along with the extended stretch, and tackling each one as it comes. This is a useful strategy for labour.

It also demonstrates that relaxation can be achieved in any position, which will be necessary and desirable in labour.

Once these extended stretches have been demonstrated in class and the concepts discussed, it's not necessary to continue practising them each week. Couples can be invited to try them at home if they wish, and this allows them to take responsibility for practice, rather than your needing to take up valuable teaching time in each class.

Points to watch

☞ There is no need to time these stretches. Indeed this is one of the important messages inherent in the exercise — that a woman has no idea how long the labour will take once it begins, and therefore worrying about time only creates a further source of anxiety. Once a contraction begins, it cannot be 'escaped' until it ends. Labour will take as long as is necessary to achieve safe arrival of the baby. By doing these stretches in this way, without an emphasis on 'contraction starting now, contraction ending now' and counting people through second by second, it is easy to illustrate the whole concept of just staying with each contraction for its duration regardless of length.

☞ If anyone, particularly a pregnant woman doing this exercise, reports pain under the rib cage (due to the size of the uterus), offer them a firm pillow to lift their buttocks a few inches off the floor. This will encourage a bend forward from the hips rather than a rounding of the back and will be more comfortable.

☞ Some people, perhaps those who are particularly anxious about pain in labour may opt out of this exercise once the initial stretch is felt. Encourage these people by using such phrases such as 'stay with it, it's still strong, it's still there, it's not going away, allow it to happen'. If you notice that there are women who regularly opt out of experiencing this extra stretch, then it may indicate a fear of pain in any form. These women may be more likely to use pain relieving drugs in labour. Individual counselling may be useful to help them confront their fears as a prelude to developing appropriate management strategies for labour.

Relaxation

As relaxation is the key to coping in labour, then it is obviously a very important topic for pre-natal classes. A relaxed state does not necessarily require a soft and floppy body: it is more centred on peace of mind, acceptance of natural processes and a willingness to embrace all that labour may offer.

Relaxation used to be taught in a very structured way in classes, with couples learning how to relax one limb while contracting all the others, and so on. This kind of disassociation drill has little relevance to labour, and does nothing to improve the mentally relaxed state of the couples in class.

Progressive relaxation exercises, perhaps incorporating imagery, are standard inclusions in stress management programs. These are valuable techniques for parents to learn for application in the post-natal period, and this should be made clear to participants. Since we are concentrating here on relaxation for labour, you will need to seek details on stress management techniques that include relaxation exercises from other sources.

Aims

✓ To explore different types of relaxation, and their uses during pregnancy, birth and the post-partum period.

✓ To explain the concept of 'automatic relaxation'.

✓ To devise strategies for encouraging automatic relaxation through the provision of a non-threatening environment, suitable human support, self-help measures and appropriate responses to painful sensations.

✓ To identify the role of the support people for a woman in labour.

✓ To assist support people to become observant of a woman's needs during labour.

✓ To develop the ability to think laterally when solving problems centred on her comfort.

✓ To encourage self-sufficiency in labour.

✓ To assist in preparing in advance for birth through choosing appropriate caregivers, place of birth, management strategies, birth options and choices.

There are many factors that affect a woman's ability to relax in labour, including:

• the physical environment

• the people in attendance, and their reactions

• the level of support from staff

• the flexibility of caregivers in meeting the woman's needs and wishes,

- the general level of trust in her ability to give birth safely
- her familiarity with the surroundings
- practical comfort measures
- the availability of non-invasive forms of pain relief
- the maintenance of her dignity and privacy
- the type of labour
- her level of pain
- fatigue, hunger and thirst
- fears and concerns about the baby
- psychological and emotional factors
- her attitudes and beliefs about labour and birth.

All of these need to be fully explored as part of the class discussion on managing labour. Some specific games and activities that enable the group to explore these issues follow. Other ideas, already mentioned, could also be adapted for teaching about relaxation.

CREATING A RELAXED ENVIRONMENT

Everyone has their own idea about what makes a particular place relaxing, comfortable and safe. Given that the physical setting plays a crucial role in the way a woman labours, identifying ways of creating the right combination of characteristics in an environment that will promote an automatic feeling of relaxation is important, particularly as women will usually be labouring in a 'foreign' environment, not normally associated with peace and privacy.

AIMS

✓ To enable group members to explore those elements that are significant in establishing an appropriate environment for labour.

✓ To encourage communication of personal needs regarding the physical and human environment in labour.

✓ To provide an opportunity for creative problem-solving.

✓ To enable expectant parents to investigate the potential birth place, and to negotiate their particular needs with caregivers.

✓ There are a number of activities that can be considered when formulating objectives for these aims:

IMAGINE A PLACE . . .

PROCESS

This is a visualisation, based on personal experience. First, the leader asks group members to close their eyes and imagine themselves in a favourite place, where they go to feel private, safe, secure and comfortable. Next, the leader asks the group to use their mind's eye, and identify the various attributes of this special place. The group can be prompted by asking key questions, to which they respond in private:

* 'How does this place look?'
* 'Is there a special colour?'
* 'How does it feel against your body?'
* 'What can you hear?'
* 'What is the temperature?'
* 'Is it light or dark?'
* 'Who is with you?'

The group members are then asked to share the answers to these questions with their partner, as a means of identifying factors that were important.

Finally, work with the partner to devise ways of establishing a similar environment in the birth place, for example: how to provide a special colour; which audiotapes would recreate significant sounds; furniture or equipment that could be adapted to provide the required level of comfort and temperature; etc.

POINTS TO WATCH

☛ It is not important that you, as leader, be told the special places recalled by the group. The important element of the exercise is to help them identify the significant factors that enhance automatic relaxation and which could be recreated in the birth place.

☛ The group may wish to share some of their findings with the larger group before moving to the problem solving part of the activity, to stimulate further thought in the group and to promote sharing.

LABOUR WARD TOURS

Visiting the labour ward is usually part of the preparation process for birth. It is useful if the tour involves the midwives in the unit, so that the women have a chance of meeting staff who may be attending them in labour. It is also helpful if the group have identified their personal needs for an appropriate environment in labour, and have already explored self-help ideas for labour and birth in their pre-natal class group. These preparatory exercises will enable them to analyse the birth area more effectively and prepare them for thinking creatively about adapting the area for their needs.

AIMS

✓ To familiarise expectant parents with the hospital setting for labour and birth.

✓ To provide an opportunity to ask questions about equipment, procedures and protocols as a basis for later negotiations with caregivers.

✓ To enable women, and their support people, to practise self-help ideas in the setting where they will be used during labour.

PROCESS

Since the labour ward tour will probably be the group's introduction to the hospital and provide the only opportunity to practise necessary skills for labour in the actual setting, the impressions gained by parents on this visit may have a critical impact on their behaviour during labour. The leader should focus primarily on the feelings engendered by the setting, and encourage group members to explore ways of adapting the setting to their own particular needs. While in the maternity unit, conducting a 'labour rehearsal' with the woman using the bean bags, mats, chairs and pillows as she may use them in labour, and having the support people find the comfort aids needed (bedpans, drinks, extra pillows, vomit bowls, extra pads etc.) will help them feel empowered through having practised in advance. Involving the staff will help give clients 'permission' to make use of the facilities, and actually using the equipment in the labour ward setting is the most effective way of promoting learning and a feeling of familiarity.

POINTS TO WATCH

☛ The emphasis should be on normal, physiological labour and how this can be achieved in the setting.

☛ Avoid focusing on the medical equipment and the bed, as this will reinforce the idea that the hospital has inflexible protocols, and a medical orientation in their management.

☛ Be sensitive to anxieties raised by the surroundings and the equipment. Avoid compounding fears by displaying frightening equipment such as forceps, needles, stirrups, fetal scalp clips for internal monitors etc. If individuals ask about this equipment, show them privately. This will avoid forcing the group to participate in a general discussion, that many may find upsetting.

☛ Address anxieties and fears by discussing how it feels to be in the room and seeing the equipment. Try to keep the discussion in perspective, through emphasising the many variations of normal birth and by not dwelling on complications and emergencies.

☛ Having participants handle basic equipment, move furniture, seek supplies and investigate drawers and cupboards is a powerful way of promoting learning and instilling confidence. It may leave the room a mess, but it will send a clear message to parents that their needs take precedence over staff needs.

'GOODY BAG'

Having inspected the hospital setting, a follow up exercise can centre on the self-help aids and supplies that the parents could take to promote comfort in labour.

AIMS

✓ To identify comfort aids for labour.

✓ To enable parents to assemble a suitable bag of 'goodies' to increase comfort and relaxation during labour.

PROCESS

This activity can be done in several ways:

- The leader supplies a drawstring bag filled with possible self-help equipment. The participants, in turn, take an item from the bag and suggest a use for it in labour. Possible inclusions in the 'goody bag' are: sponge, wash cloth, water spray, sweets, a drink, sandwich or packet of dried fruit (or some other suitable food items), music tape, magazine, shower hat, slippers, large T-shirt, cloth nappy (diaper) and a pair of rubber gloves, warm socks, etc.
- The leader passes around a large sheet of butcher's paper and the participants either list or draw a contribution to the goody bag, explaining the reason for their choice.
- The leader can display the contents of the goody bag and invite the participants to choose comfort aids to practise with during a labour rehearsal or whilst experimenting with positions for labour and birth.
- Following on from these activities, the participants can devise their own personal list, perhaps working with their partner.

POINTS TO WATCH

- ☛ The support people have a need for comfort aids in labour as well as the mother. Attention needs to be paid to including appropriate items for them as well.
- ☛ Using equipment such as pretend hot packs and hot, wet nappies during labour rehearsals is an effective way to familiarise participants with their use and to enhance leaning.

POSITIONS

Learning how to increase comfort and aid dilatation through appropriate positioning during labour is a basic element of active birth classes. This is a broad and extensive topic, deserving of several practice sessions.

AIMS

- ✓ To enable group members to explore ways of increasing the comfort of the labouring woman.
- ✓ To provide insight into the needs of women in labour.
- ✓ To assist support people develop sensitivity to the labouring woman's needs and to promote their powers of observation.
- ✓ To provide an opportunity for creative problem solving.

PROCESS

This topic could be broken into two or three practice sessions: early first stage of labour, transition, and second stage (followed briefly by third stage).

The leader suggests various scenarios to the group, who are then encouraged to work with a partner to make her comfortable. For example:

- an aching back
- heavy pressure in the lower abdomen
- the need to rest her legs
- pressure in the vulval area
- getting comfortable on a bedpan or on the toilet etc.

As the support teams organise the chairs, pillows, bean bags etc. to meet her pretend needs, the woman provides feedback on their efforts. The leader circulates to assist with any special problems (stiff knees, bad backs etc.). When everyone has found a useful posture, the leader uses the group members to demonstrate possible solutions. The group then tries ideas they have observed other people using.

POINTS TO WATCH

- ☛ In the first session where positions are practised, group members may feel a little embarrassed or inhibited. Try dimming the lights or providing some background music to enhance a feeling of privacy (and provide additional learning points for later use in labour wards).

- ☛ Avoid demonstrating positions to the group for them to copy. This removes the element of problem solving, and discourages participants from taking responsibility for their own needs. It may also create the idea that certain positions are preferable or 'correct' since they have been demonstrated by the leader when, in reality, any position is fine, as long as it is comfortable for the woman.

- ☛ Remind the class of appropriate physiology already discussed, for example, that remaining upright maintains the pressure of the baby on the cervix which keeps the contractions efficient and regular.

- ☛ Use examples from everyday life when appropriate: it is quite possible to fall asleep sitting in a chair provided you are well supported, so this can be adapted in labour for when she is tired, without resorting to lying down, which tends to slow labour and make it more uncomfortable.

- ☛ Provide a variety of pillows, bean bags, chairs and mats that can be used and adapted as necessary. Avoid using a bed or suggesting recumbent positions. This is especially important in second stage, when taking to a bed significantly reduces the options available to a woman for choosing various physiologic positions.

☛ Emphasise that being creative, thinking laterally and learning to be adaptive are important elements of this exercise. Making the most of the equipment you have is essential when labour takes place in restrictive or 'foreign' environments.

☛ Reinforcing the learning through providing a follow up session in the actual hospital labour ward (as part of the tour) is a valuable way of empowering people to use the ideas when the time comes.

MASSAGE, TOUCH AND OTHER SELF HELP STRATEGIES

These self-help measures can be incorporated into the practice sessions on positions for labour and birth. In this way their relevance, and their appropriate use, will be more readily learned and remembered by support people.

AIMS

✓ To encourage self-reliance during labour, and creative problem-solving in the support team for a labouring woman.

✓ To explore various comfort measures and their application during labour.

PROCESS

Practice in using these measures can become an additional element in labour rehearsals. There are a number of 'hands-on' activities that can be included: massage, effleurage, sacral pressure, hot packs, and showers and baths.

MASSAGE

Massage techniques need to be kept simple as most support people, particularly the fathers, have little experience of massage and are not necessarily adept at learning it at this stage in the pregnancy. The most important element of massage is the touching and close contact that is provided by this technique, and as long as the mother feels free to give feedback about the effect of the massage, then usually some appropriate measures will be devised during labour. When discussing and demonstrating massage, it is vital to show the person doing the massage how to position themselves to avoid fatigue or potential problems with their own back.

Show them how to kneel with one knee up, as shown, or how to stand with one foot in front of the other. This will allow free movement through the legs without stress to their backs (figure 27).

When applying sacral pressure to relieve backache, use both hands, as shown above, to increase the comfort of the support person and provide sufficient

FIGURE 27

Kneeling like this, with one leg up, will protect the support person's back while massaging.

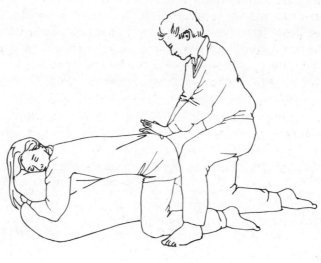

FIGURE 28

Long strokes down the back can be soothing.

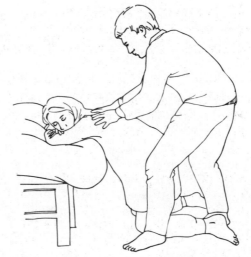

FIGURE 29

Pressure on the shoulders relieves tension.

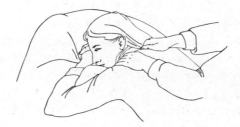

pressure. Remember that the sore point on the mother's back will be quite localised and may move through labour as the baby turns and descends, and that feedback from her will be essential to get the pressure positioned correctly. Keep the elbows straight and bend the knees to allow the body weight of the support person to be transferred to her back. Use plenty of cushioning under the mother's knees and keep her back parallel to the floor, with her knees under her hips for maximal effect (figure 28).

Long strokes using the palm of the hand and relaxed fingers down each side of the spine are very soothing, particularly in between contractions during a long backache labour. Continuing the hands down over the buttocks and the tops of the thighs lengthens the stroke and provides comfort to an area that is often carrying considerable tension throughout labour.

Effleurage is a light fingertip stroking over the tummy and can be particularly useful to relieve pain. Very gentle stroking is all that is required, and by reaching around under her tummy this can be done with the mother in any upright position.

Holding is a very simple technique that helps to calm a woman who is showing signs of distress. It is particularly useful in transition. The support person places their hands over the tops of the shoulders, and applies gentle but firm downward pressure (figure 29).

Make sure that the thumbs are not gripping the shoulders. Putting your arms around someone and holding them in this way can have a very calming effect on a woman who is feeling particularly out of control through a turbulent transition. Similar holding around the hips can also be comforting.

Face massage — a gentle stroking — can be useful to provide overall relief and relaxation during labour. Gentle stroking of the brow, of the area on either side of the eyes, and of the jaw and chin, will help to remind a woman to release tension in those areas (figure 30).

Foot massage, particularly in a long labour, can provide immeasurable relief. The feet often become quite cold in labour, and the mother may enjoy having warm hands applied to her feet and the application of some gentle kneading and stroking. If she is ticklish, use firm pressure (figure 31).

HEAT AND WATER

A combination of heat and water can be a most effective form of pain relief for many women in labour. The relaxing effects of getting into a hot bath are well known to most people, and are therefore easily visualised. Many hospitals are not equipped with a bath, and so some alternative form of heat and water (the shower and hot packs of various types) can be used instead. A woman using the shower during labour still needs company and support so it is useful for

FIGURE 30

*Massaging
the face can be
comforting.*

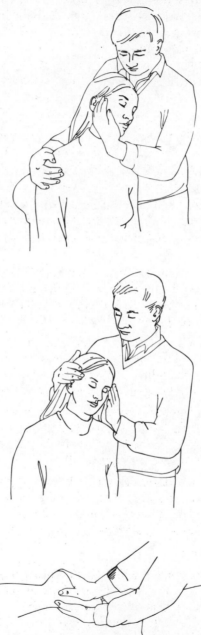

FIGURE 31

*Firm
pressure on
the feet
provides
warmth.*

couples to practise providing assistance and comfort in simulated conditions. There should be a stool or chair in the shower cubicle that can be used to sit or lean on, and extra towels on the floor will relieve pressure on the knees.

Hot packs come in various forms, either jelly-filled or sand-filled (hydrocolater units). The latter provide limited assistance — their main disadvantage is that they are hard to position and are heavy. They do, however, retain their heat for a considerable time and so are useful as a source of localised heat in certain circumstances.

The simplest form of providing water and heat is to use hot, wet nappies or towels. The necessary equipment should be taken to the hospital so that it will be available when needed. Two or three nappies, a large pair of rubber gloves, and a bucket will be required. The water needs to be very hot as it will cool rapidly, even when the bucket is almost full of water. The towels should be wrung out so that they are not dripping, and then be applied over whatever area is most in need. They can also be overlapped all down her back and over her buttocks, or she might choose to have them folded up and positioned over the vulva or against her lower abdomen. Because wringing out towels for extended periods is exhausting for the support person, it is helpful to save this form of pain relief until transition when it will be most appreciated. Pretending to use these hot packs or towels can form part of the labour rehearsal and the actual equipment can be supplied as part of the leader's goody bag.

LABOUR REHEARSALS

A review session where all the skills and suggestions for ensuring comfort, privacy and automatic relaxation for a woman in labour are brought together can be valuable to cement learning and increase feelings of confidence and competence. This session would need to be scheduled towards the end of the class series, but with sufficient time afterwards to recap on information or reinforce particular skills if needed.

Since it is impossible to predict how labour will eventuate, your group will need to practise in hypothetical situations, in a way that is non-threatening, particularly when preparing for possible complications or variations.

AIMS

✓ To provide a review session and summary of the skills and information learned through the class series.

✓ To provide a practical session to build feelings of confidence and competence in the expectant mother and her support team.

✓ To encourage the use of problem-solving techniques that can be useful in labour.

✓ To enable group members to explore pregnancy, labour, birth and the first hours post-partum as a continuum.

PROCESS

Labour rehearsals can be stages in several ways:

SITUATION ('WHAT IF?') CARDS

A set of cards is prepared, each containing the outline of a scenario during labour. Each woman in the group selects a card (this reinforces the idea that anything can occur in labour) and works with her partner and support people to formulate answers to two questions: 'What may be happening here?' and 'What could be done about it?' Each card is read out and the answers are shared with the large group. Further input from others may be invited and comment from the leader can also be added.

POINTS TO WATCH

☞ Choose scenarios that are likely to occur. For example, if local hospital policy states that on admission, a 20 minute baseline trace using an electronic fetal monitor will be taken, include this scenario on a card, to enable the group to explore their options in this situation. This allows you to present likely situations in an ethical manner, and to equip group members with specific skills that may be useful. Many report afterwards that they were surprised how labour turned out to be 'Just like on that card you gave us!' This kind of rehearsal can be very empowering as it focuses on behaviours, feelings and reactions as well as practical techniques.

☛ Write the scenarios in the third person rather than the first person. Finding a solution for a problem faced by 'Mary', 'Jane' or 'Joan' is less threatening than being confronted by the situation 'You have just . . .' or 'You are . . .'

☛ Prepare scenarios that are open ended, that is, where more than one solution to the problem is possible. This encourages lateral thinking.

☛ If information is needed, or it becomes apparent that vital facts have been overlooked, you should include them and correct any misinterpretations. you could also invite the group to propose questions that could be asked to clarify a situation, and extend this to include discussion on the language and phrasing that might be used.

ROLE PLAYING

Practising the management of various situations in life, as an actual rehearsal, can be used to develop skills and build of confidence. Role plays can evolve from the situation cards described above or can be arranged as a separate activity.

AIMS

✓ To allow participants to get first hand experience in a given situation.
✓ To enable players to see a situation from another person's point of view, which is useful when negotiation is necessary.
✓ To practise specific skills as a confidence building exercise.

PROCESS

The participants can either choose their own scenario and prepare a script or a situation can be presented to the group, perhaps using a prepared script or background notes (such as a situation card).

The group members adopt appropriate roles. Playing themselves allows participants to explore personal feelings, reactions and behaviours, whilst playing someone else promotes insight and understanding of another's position and behaviours.

The group rehearses if necessary, then acts out the scene. Those watching observe the behaviours, language, reactions and results of the player's involvement. Feedback is sought, from the players ('How was it when . . . said to you?', 'What was it like finding yourself . . .?', 'What would you have liked to happen when . . .?') and from the observers ('What did you notice when . . .?', 'What were the feelings of the various players?').

The scene is re-enacted to effect a different, more desirable outcome, using modifications as decided by the group or suggested by the leader. Feedback is again sought, focusing on the differences felt by the players on this second occasion.

Several scenarios may be acted out in this way. At the end of the session, the whole group discusses the value of role play, what they have discovered, how they might use the information gained etc.

POINTS TO WATCH

☛ Many people find role plays threatening and uncomfortable. Either call for volunteers, or allow people to invoke the 'right to pass' group rule if they wish. You need to explain the advantages of role playing, the benefits of practising responses in this way, and that you are not judging acting ability! If you have established a supportive and co-operative group, role play can be useful and fun, and provide an unmatched opportunity for participants to explore various issues directly.

☛ Allow people time to get into role, and to step out of their role afterwards. Choosing character's names that are different from their own, or wearing name tags with titles (e.g. the doctor, midwife, mother, father) helps players to separate themselves from the role and to be more objective.

☛ When giving feedback, always use the character's name or title, and never the actual player's name.

☛ Role playing is time consuming. If you try to rush through a role play, the benefits will be lost. If time is limited, choose another activity.

'DEMONSTRATING' LABOUR

Another way of presenting a role play is to demonstrate labour behaviours yourself.

AIMS

✓ To allow group members to explore the feelings associated with watching someone in 'labour'.

✓ To present possible behaviour patterns as a means of preparing support people and the women themselves, for potential reactions in labour.

PROCESS

Select someone from the group to be your 'support person' during the demonstration. This should be done prior to the session with enough time to develop a plan of action for the demonstration.

Explain to the group that you will demonstrate a typical contraction. Transition offers lots of scope!

Position yourself with appropriate props, and play act the contraction showing your reactions as the support person fulfils their previously discussed role.

After the contraction ends, allow a few moments for recovery, then initiate a discussion about the demonstration: what was observed, how people felt watching it, what they would have liked to do, etc.

Follow up with a discussion on the merits of the activity, and elaborate further using videos or audiotapes if you wish.

POINTS TO WATCH

☞ Some people may become quite upset watching a contraction like this, particularly without the foregoing labour to accustom them to a variety of responses. This issue needs to be discussed.

☞ Acting out contractions in this way is a useful way of addressing the emotional reactions of support people in labour, and their need for support. In introducing this discussion point, a lead-in activity such as 'sentence stems' could be used.

AUDIO AND VIDEO TAPES

Audio or video tapes can also be used to present information and initiate discussion about physiological birth and the management of labour. They can be used to either open a session, followed by discussion, or to summarise discussion at the close of a session. Video tapes need to be chosen with great care, and there is more information on how to do this in Part 4.

AIMS

✓ To provide an alternative means of presenting information on labour and birth in a realistic form.

✓ To present a variety of labours to the group, so that the various responses and management techniques used can be explored in depth.

✓ To stimulate discussion on the role of the support person, the reactions of women during labour and the specific techniques, procedures and interventions available during labour.

✓ To demonstrate some of the options and choices available to labouring women.

PROCESS

A video or audio tape is selected, and presented either wholly or in part. The tape may be stopped at any time for discussion or to explain what is happening. After it has finished, and a few moments have been allowed for quiet reflection, the leader initiates a discussion, either highlighting particular issues raised by the tape, or to elicit feelings and reactions of the group to the presentation.

POINTS TO WATCH

☛ It is hard to predict group members' reactions to audio or video tapes. Be prepared for any response, and use appropriate counselling responses to further the conversation.

☛ It is not necessary to show the entire video, particularly if time is short, or if you wish to highlight certain parts. The group will probably want to know how the labour ended, so either show the birth later or give full details of the eventual outcome.

☛ try to show several labour videos to avoid creating the impression that there is only one way to labour, and to demonstrate choice during a variety of births.

Exploring choice

Most childbirth educators would state that informed choice is a basic corner-stone of preparation for parenthood classes. They believe that well informed people will be better able to make necessary decisions during labour and birth and will be more satisfied afterwards, having been fully involved throughout labour. At post-natal reunions, as parents recount the lists of interventions that so often occur during birth, educators may wonder whether all the time and effort spent in giving people the facts was really worthwhile.

Making an informed decision is more than knowing the options, advantages, disadvantages and alternatives. It takes skills and perseverance, plus commit-ment, to be successful in having your needs met, especially in a system where it is the caregiver(s) who have traditionally made all the decisions, without consulting or even considering (in many cases) the wishes and desires of their clients.

Therefore, if women and their partners are to be truly empowered to have an active birth, enabling parents to acquire the skills necessary to achieve their goals for birth is probably the most important aspect of your teaching. These are not skills centred on learning birthing behaviours (women already have those) but rather those that help parents to use the health care system to their best advantage. The medicalisation of birth has presented parents with a bewildering array of choices and options: finding a way through this maze forces parents to confront dilemmas, decisions that need to be made, opportu-nities for negotiation, and a mass of information that needs to be sifted, sorted and interpreted. Activities in pre-natal classes that practise dealing with these can assist parents to be better prepared for facing these important issues that surround birth.

Aims

We will have a number of aims in addressing these areas of concern, includ-ing:

✓ To provide opportunities for parents to practise making decisions, negoti-ating options and exercising choice.

✓ To explore emotions and feelings associated with these processes.

✓ To enable parents to identify issues surrounding birth that have personal significance and importance.

✓ To encourage parents to develop flexible, open attitudes to the potential outcomes of birth.

PROCESS

Every activity in your pre-natal class series should have an objective that enables one or more of these aims to be met. In other words, the skills and competencies outlined above are applicable to almost every topic in your class series, and this theme of consumerism can be woven into every topic in some way. Instead of presenting a session on 'making choices' or 'becoming assertive', try to plan all your teaching strategies to incorporate an objective on decision-making and problem solving. This will offer parents many occasions in which to practise these skills. There are a number of possible activities:

BRAINSTORMING

This is a useful step in creative problem solving, which can be incorporated into other activities where the group needs to identify potential solutions in hypothetical situations.

AIMS

✓ To encourage lateral thinking.
✓ To expose members to other ways of thinking about or perceiving a situation.
✓ To boost the energy in the group.

PROCESS

The leader presents a topic to the group and invites spontaneous 'off the top of the head' comments. All comments are recorded and displayed. The group then discusses the range of comments, and is invited to make observations on what has been revealed.

It may be appropriate to use their list as a basis for agenda setting, or for prioritising issues to be discussed later.

POINTS TO WATCH

☞ This activity is generally used to help participants move into an expansionary frame of mind, with the accent on finding positive suggestions. If the group begins to focus on negative responses, draw their attention to what is happening, and ask them to balance their negative comments with positive ones.

DISCUSSION

Since there will be many individual situations amongst the group members to explore, discussion and sharing ideas is worthwhile.

AIMS

✓ To share strategies for making decisions.

✓ To explore the concept of choice and the range of potential circumstances where choices can be made.

✓ To canvass resources useful in the process of making a decision.

✓ To provide information, on request, that may be helpful for clients.

PROCESS

IN EARLY PREGNANCY CLASSES

- How did you choose your midwife or doctor?
- Do you know what tests have been ordered for you?
- What were the results of these tests?
- Have you chosen a birth place as yet?
- How to make the most of pre-natal visits with your caregiver
- How to get a second medical opinion, and how to change doctors, if desired

IN PARENTING CLASSES

- Community resources for parents
- Choosing baby care equipment
- Breast or bottle feeding
- Sharing the household tasks
- Choosing child care etc.

IN BIRTH CLASSES

- Options for management of late pregnancy complications
- Labour ward tours
- Induction issues
- Negotiating labour management with caregivers: positions for birth, pain relief options, using the bath or shower (water birth?), oxytocics for third stage, etc.
- Birth outcomes: sick babies, handicaps, stillbirth
- Post natal issues: circumcision, Vitamin K, unrestricted breastfeeding, etc.

The discussion can be initiated and managed in several ways — please refer to the suggestions on page 137.

POINTS TO WATCH

☞ Be aware of your own position on these issues, to avoid instilling bias into the discussion.

☞ Encourage the group to explore all options, even if some may not be readily available in the hospitals they have chosen. If you present only those services provided in these maternity units or only mention the management options preferred by the local practitioners, consumers will not be aware of the full range of options available to them. If they decide that an issue is of such importance that it merits looking beyond the local services, then parents can decide what they want to do: accept the current position, go elsewhere, or stay and negotiate some changes.

☞ Many people, particularly pregnant women, fear changing doctors because of the possible social ramifications, especially if they live in a close knit community or small town. You will need to help them explore their personal feelings, and perhaps assist them to deal with these issues directly with the people concerned. Your support may be crucial in enabling them to make changes in their maternity care.

☞ You will need to be resourceful. Having a list of useful local services for parents, knowing the health services available in the area and elsewhere, and being able to suggest health practitioners for special needs should all be part of your service as an educator.

☞ Many educators fear ethical dilemmas that may arise during discussion on consumer issues, and avoid introducing the topic. Provided that you are giving facts, are not presenting a personal view or giving advice, ethical dilemmas should not be a problem. If you are confronted by your colleagues, or challenged to explain what you have been discussing in class, you will need to deal with this assertively. Parents have a right to information, and providing this, in a fair and understandable manner, is part to your job description. Some parents misinterpret your statements or comments, however, and this is often at the heart of the conflict. Finding solutions to these situations is an important element in your own development as an educator, and can be a useful experience in developing strategies for teaching.

BIRTH GUIDELINES

Parents are often encouraged in class to develop a 'wish' list of what they would like to have happen during the birth.

Aims

✓ To identify those issues that are especially important or significant for women during labour and birth.

✓ To use this list as a basis for communication and negotiation with caregivers.

✓ To canvass the wide range of possible outcomes of labour and birth.

✓ To ensure that parents have considered their options as a basis for making an informed decision, as part of the consent process.

The preparation by your clients of a statement of preferences or guidelines for labour, birth and the post-partum period often forms a focal point in the discussion on consumerism in childbirth. These statements need to:

- be broadly written, not narrowly constructed,
- allow for changes to be made, as necessary, at all times and especially during the birth process,
- avoid being prescriptive, e.g. 'I wish to choose my own birth position', rather than 'I want to squat',
- provide for the unexpected, perhaps by stating 'I wish to be consulted on all decisions',
- be clear in their intent, without being emotional,
- be simple and concise, not lengthy or rambling.

Process

The uses of birth guidelines can be introduced into the group at any appropriate time. Some educators like to use them as a running theme, commenting on topics that could be included in a guideline at various points in the class.

The most important element in the discussion on birth guidelines, however, is to formulate procedures for implementing the ideas it contains. In order to obtain the care they feel is important, parents may need to negotiate on various points, or seek second opinions, even change caregivers. These possibilities can be discussed or even practised in class, using role plays, situation cards, visits to the maternity unit, inviting guests (caregivers, new parents) to the class to present their experiences, viewing videos etc.

Points to watch

☞ Some parents become so engrossed in preparing the perfect birth 'plan' that they fail to consider alternatives, and the uncontrollable nature of labour and birth. A narrow focus and dogmatic ideas can lead to great disappointment and grief when events unfold in a different way from what was expected. This is an issue that needs to be canvassed, perhaps as part of the theme of dealing with unexpected outcomes.

☛ Be aware of your own personal experiences, and avoid setting people up to copy you. A leader is a powerful role model in this situation, and you should stay alert to any of your own biases that may accidentally creep into the discussion. Avoid using your own birth experiences as examples.

SHOPPING FOR SERVICES

AIMS

✓ To provide information about the services available in the community.

✓ To encourage parents to seek their own information from community service representatives.

✓ To introduce a number of resource personnel to the group at one time, without taking up valuable class time with a series of individual visits.

PROCESS

This can be a fun way of introducing the idea of choice into selecting services, particularly for birth and parenting.

The educator arranges a 'market night' (or a similar title), and invites representatives of local service providers to attend. Each representative is given a table to display information, goods or services and is invited to speak to group members, who are free to move around between the displays. Services that could be included are:

- community health centre
- early childhood clinic
- local doctors
- independent midwives
- community support groups (for breastfeeding mothers, parents of handicapped babies, single mothers etc.)
- baby care equipment retailers
- child safety officer
- nutritionist
- massage therapist
- swimming or aerobics classes for new mothers (or any other recreational activity)
- first aid officer etc.

This is a particularly useful activity for larger groups of parents, and encourages them to 'shop around'. It is also a way of avoiding the disruption to group dynamics of having guests visit the classes individually.

POINTS TO WATCH

☞ It will take some time to organise the initial market night. You will need enough space, and tables for your visitors to display their materials. Allow time for setting up and for the parents to circulate.

☞ This event could also be used as a way of attracting clients to your classes, if it was advertised to a wider audience, perhaps through the local media. It could be arranged as a regular event for the local community.

☞ A thank-you note to each visitor following the market night would be a thoughtful gesture, which would encourage participation another time.

VISITS BY NEW PARENTS

AIMS

✓ To provide an opportunity for expectant parents to meet some new parents with their babies.

✓ To enable parents to see what a newborn baby is like, and perhaps to view some basic baby care in action.

✓ To encourage new and expectant parents to discuss parenting experiences, including the birth and the early days following the baby's arrival.

✓ To bring some realism into the class!

Having new parents visit the class with their new baby provides an opening for discussion on a range of topics:

- birth experiences,
- unexpected outcomes,
- labour and birth options,
- care of the new baby,
- breastfeeding,
- family adjustments and changing lifestyles etc.

PROCESS

The educator invites one or more new parents to visit the current pre-natal class group.

The visitors are invited to tell their story, and the group can ask questions. You may also like to ask questions, to open up the conversation, to help the new parents focus on key issues, and to keep the session moving forward.

Following the visit, the group will need time to debrief, and to discuss their responses to the story they have just heard.

POINTS TO WATCH

☛ In selecting these visitors, there is no need to choose only those who have had 'good' births or parents who are happy with their birth outcome. The main criteria in choosing these guests are: a willingness to attend the group; an ability to speak to others and share their experiences; and being reasonably well adjusted to their changed circumstances and the birth outcome.

☛ Schedule the visit at a time to suit the new parents. Be aware that the baby will become the focus of attention, and that your input, as leader, will be very limited!

☛ Discuss with the visiting mother, before she arrives, how she feels about breastfeeding in front of the group should this be necessary, and also performing other basic baby care, such as nappy changing. These can be valuable for your group to witness, and can lead to useful discussion.

☛ Try to limit the visit to a suitable length. New parents don't want to be kept up late at night, and you must allow time to debrief after they have left. Scheduling a coffee break immediately after the visit allows time for the visitors to depart and the group to reform.

☛ If the visitors embark on a tale of woe, be ready to help them seek the positive aspects of their experience. A question such as 'What did you discover from this?', 'What was the best part of the event?' or 'How would you change things another time?' can lead to consideration of more positive outcomes. All stories have the potential to make group members anxious, and this is the reason why careful debriefing is necessary afterwards.

DEALING WITH THE UNEXPECTED

It is impossible to prepare people for unexpected outcomes, since there is no way of predicting what these outcomes may be, and therefore no way of anticipating how people will react or feel. In addition, focusing on what can go wrong invites people to make predictions about the future, and this can lead to self-fulfilling prophecies and negative thinking.

How can we help clients keep an open mind about future events, yet feel prepared to deal with unexpected outcomes? Teaching strategies that focus on analysing past experiences to identify what may have been helpful in other unexpected situations is one way. Another is to use analogies to focus on the concept that life is unpredictable, and that sometimes these unforeseen and even unwelcome outcomes can have positive effects on individuals.

LIFE SO FAR . . .

This activity is designed to help participants identify the mechanisms they have used in the past to deal with unexpected events.

AIMS

✓ To enable participants to identify major life events that have had a major impact in their lives.

✓ To identify both the positive and negative learning outcomes to be gained from these events.

✓ To compile a list of personal resources available in the event of need.

PROCESS

Each individual is given a sheet of paper and a pencil. The leader invites everyone to remember an experience they have had that was unexpected, and which had an impact on their lives. Explain that this event will not be revealed to the group, but kept private.

Each person then makes a list of the aspects of this experience they found to be positive, negative and interesting, and what they learned from it.

In either small groups, or the large group, members then share their findings, without revealing their personal life-shaping event. The results can be recorded on butcher's paper or a whiteboard and displayed for all to see. The leader then compiles or highlights the personal resources mentioned by group members, that could be used again in the future.

POINTS TO WATCH

☛ Good leadership skills will be required for this exercise.

☛ Try to ensure that participants don't reveal their personal life events. It is more important to concentrate on the effects this experience had rather than the event itself. The group may become bogged down in someone's traumatic story rather than focusing on the skills and resources that were gained.

☛ Keep the group thinking of positives. If necessary, initiate the identification of positives by asking question such as '. . . and what did you gain from this?', 'How did this help you in the end?', 'What did you find useful in these circumstances?'

☛ When summarising the skills gained by members of the group stress that something positive can be gained from every life event, and that resources, both internal and external, are available in case of need.

ANALOGIES AND STORY TELLING

Storytelling and analogies can be used to explore concepts and help participants maintain big picture perspectives, useful in times of crises.

AIMS

✓ To provide an opportunity to explore the unexpected nature of life events.

✓ To enable parents to examine major life events and their impact without direct personal involvement, since the events relate to others, not themselves.

PROCESS

The leader reads an appropriate story and then invites comment on the meaning of the story, and what its message is in relation to birth or parenting. Excerpts from novels, birth or parenting stories may be used. Choosing stories with a cultural significance may be useful for some groups.

Analogies can be constructed by the leader, or examples drawn from novels, written narratives etc. Some examples:

LABOUR AND BIRTH IS A LITTLE LIKE GOING ON HOLIDAY

Choosing a holiday location (deciding on what you want); planning an appropriate time to go; deciding how to travel to the destination (direct, by the scenic route, by car, train or plane); what to take for the journey (companions, food, maps etc.); taking your time on the trip or going directly (stop overs, seeing the sights, going by the shortest, fastest route); the inability to prepare for the road surface, road works, pilot's strikes etc. (depending on your mode of travel); the unexpected along the way (car sickness, minor accidents, getting lost etc.); and the final arrival (does the destination live up to expectations?). Would you go again? How would you travel next time? etc.

Becoming a parent has similarities to getting your first job

Training for the task as best you can, not knowing exactly what is required; making your application; preparing for the interview; being given the job; finding that it differs from the job description; discovering that your training wasn't enough to ensure instant competence; trying to learn on-the-job; dealing with the stresses of the job; trying to match the expectations of the boss (especially if your boss is rather uncommunicative); trying to be as good as everyone else; gradually feeling more competent; finally feeling comfortable; being able to assist others in turn; applying for a higher position; taking on more responsibility . . .

The difference between spontaneous labour and induction could be likened to two ways of learning to swim

The gradual approach — trying out the water; moving into deeper water; getting the idea of how to stay afloat; learning how to move your arms to make progress; finally reaching the pontoon or end of the pool using your own efforts.

The 'sink-or-swim method' — being taken to the pool or out to the pontoon in a boat; being thrown into water over your head; being either left to learn quickly or given assistance (a lifeline, a float to take you over the water to the other side) or rescue (a boat to lift you out altogether).

The stages of labour are similar to driving up a hill

Cruising along the flat with the hill and its lookout in the distance; taking the small foothills in one's stride; needing to change down a gear for the slightly higher slopes; a low gear and careful negotiation around the steep hair-pin bends near the top; reaching the look out, seeing where you have driven from (and seeing what lies ahead!).

Choosing caregivers is like selecting a tradesman to do some plumbing

Compiling a list of local tradesman; deciding on the work to be done; preparing a list of specifications; interviewing possible plumbers — asking for recommendations, inspecting previous work, discussing costs, availability, preferred way of tackling the work etc.; engaging the tradesman; supervising his work; making changes as needed; evaluating the job; recommending him to others.

CHOOSING AN OBSTETRICIAN COULD BE LIKENED TO BUYING STORM AND TEMPEST INSURANCE FOR YOUR HOME

Deciding you need insurance; shopping around for the best deal; paying the premium; feeling secure knowing you have the insurance if the roof blows off; calling the insurance company when the roof does blow away in a freak storm; assessing how much repair work is needed; getting the work done; feeling pleased the insurance was available!

POINTS TO WATCH

☛ Being prepared to do some acting, and to inject humour and interest into a story. Good use of vocabulary, and choosing culturally appropriate words and language will help.

☛ There is no need to necessarily draw a moral from an analogy or story. Listeners can be left to draw their own conclusions, commenting if they wish.

☛ Keep it short to avoid becoming boring!

☛ Use analogies and stories sparingly or they may lose their impact.

IN THE EVENT THAT . . .

AIMS

✓ To describe the services available to parents in the event of a premature birth, stillbirth, handicapped baby etc.

✓ To provide information about the kinds of reactions that may be experienced.

✓ To allow discussion of these fears, often felt by parents during pregnancy.

PROCESS

Group discussion is possibly the most effective way to raise this topic. Try to lead into the discussion as a natural follow on from another topic, rather than introducing it 'cold'. It is important to obtain permission from the group before proceeding. Following introductory remarks covering the main points, you may wish to invite group members to share any experiences they have had with these kinds of outcomes. Discussion should focus on the inability to be prepared for these kinds of events; the need to be aware of the many physical and emotional reactions that may result, all of which are normal; the services and resources that are available if needed; and the answering of specific questions posed by the group members.

POINTS TO WATCH

☞ Keep the discussion contained (avoid long, sad accounts) and try to present the topic at a time when it can be followed by something positive or fun.

☞ Acknowledging people's feelings will be helpful — 'It is hard to talk about these subjects. However, I think we should take a few minutes to consider . . .', 'I find it really hard to talk about these kinds of outcomes, but I guess it is something we should consider', 'I think we need to move on to something more cheerful now'.

☞ Avoid giving reassurances — 'I'm sure none of you will have to face these problems', 'This is unlikely to happen to you' etc. They sound hollow and are unrealistic. Adults can often tell when they are being fobbed off, and if you fail to acknowledge their fears in this area, you risk appearing unconcerned, or frightened of these topics yourself, which will lower your credibility.

☞ Be honest about your own feelings if necessary, as this can help group rapport.

☞ Avoid initiating this discussion just before the close of the session. If it arises late in the class, take extra time to finish and to send people off in a positive mood. Never fob off discussion by holding it over to the next session. It is important to deal with feelings in this area immediately they arise.

TEACHING ABOUT DRUGS AND INTERVENTIONS

It is important to include factual information in your class on all the potential drugs, medical procedures and obstetric complications so that your clients can use the information when they are making decisions. This can be a difficult area to cover since it tends to be a 'heavy' topic, couched in medical terms, and centres on topics many people would rather avoid, such as forceps and caesareans.

AIMS

✓ To provide background information that parents will find useful when making decisions.

✓ To ensure that parents are well informed when being asked for their consent to interventions in birth.

✓ To correct and myths and misinformation expressed by group members.

PROCESS

This can be a complex, difficult topic so try to avoid dealing with all the complications, drugs and obstetric procedures in one session. Instead, include each one when discussing the relevant stage of pregnancy or labour, and balance it with information on uncomplicated birth and self help measures etc. For example:

THE LAST WEEKS OF PREGNANCY

- pre-eclampsia
- persistent breech
- premature birth

BEGINNING LABOUR

- induction
- prostaglandins

EARLY FIRST STAGE

- when to go to hospital
- admission procedures — electronic fetal monitoring, enemas, shaving
- artificial rupture of membranes

MID FIRST STAGE

- oxytocin drips for slow labour
- pain relieving drugs for induced births — pethidine

Late first stage (transition)

- epidurals, nitrous oxide
- fetal distress
- caesarean section

Second stage

- forceps
- vacuum extraction
- episiotomy
- pudendal blocks, local anaesthetics

Third stage

- oxytocics for third stage
- perineal repair

When presenting factual information, especially in the form of a lecturette, it is important to maintain the group's interest and make sure that they are receiving the message. In particular, be aware of:

- Your language — avoid jargon, aim for simple explanations. Avoid being overly dramatic, or underplaying the seriousness of the topic through your choice of words.

- Personal bias — often conveyed through your choice of words. Avoid words with emotional overtones, try to keep the discussion neutral.

- Non-verbal cues — the look on your face, your tone of voice, the emphasis you place on certain words or events, may all reveal a personal point of view that may distort your message or impose an opinion that may affect other people's judgement or decisions.

- The amount of time allocated to these subjects — try to keep balance and perspective between the normal and the complications in labour.

- The feelings these topics engender in others — most people are fearful of complications, and many have heard alarming stories about births that went wrong. Take note of the reactions in your group, and where they occur. Find a way to address these feelings and emotional reactions as part of the discussion.

Of course, it is essential that you are fully aware of the facts as they relate to these complications and that you present a balanced picture of the advantages and disadvantages of intervention so that truly informed choice can be made. Make sure you are up-to-date with the latest scientific findings on the effects of drugs and technology in birth and revise your presentation as often as necessary. Sometimes this may mean altering your own personal views as well, as new scientific facts come to light.

To assist in presenting the full picture, it can be helpful to carry a mental 'game plan' in your head, to work through with each topic:

- A brief description of the procedure, drug or intervention
- Indications for its use
- How it is administered
- Effects on the mother — advantages and disadvantages
- Effects on the baby — advantages and disadvantages
- Alternatives, when available.

Once you have presented the group with the factual information about these issues, it is possible to introduce activities that help to re-enforce the facts, deal with the emotional issues that surround them and explore attitudes to their use. Some of these activities can also form the basis of an evaluation, to help you make sure that group members have grasped the relevant points and understand the reasons for and implications of obstetric interventions.

SORT THE FACTS

This is a simple card game that enables the group to demonstrate their understanding of the facts relating to drugs or procedures.

AIMS

✓ To review information given earlier.
✓ To assess the level of understanding of the issues being presented.
✓ To provide an alternative means of presenting technical information, other than a lecturette.

PROCESS

The leader prepares a set of cards, each one stating a fact that relates to the issues being addressed. For example, to explore the use of drugs for pain relief, there would need to be three sets of cards, for epidural, pethidine, and nitrous oxide and oxygen. The epidural set has statements such as 'slows second stage', 'usually provides full pain relief', 'restricts mobility' etc. Similar statements are assembled for the other drugs.

The leader places the three drug title cards on the floor, then asks each group member to choose a card at random from the pack of statement cards. These are then placed under the appropriate heading. Discussion follows, and, if needed, any corrections are made or additional information is provided.

CASCADE OF INTERVENTIONS

A variation on the above game, to help group members grasp the links between one intervention and the other.

AIMS

✓ To help reinforce the information that one intervention in labour may lead to another.

✓ To summarise the information on drugs and interventions.

✓ To evaluate the group's level of understanding of the issues surrounding the use of drugs and technology during birth.

PROCESS

The leader prepares a time line of labour and birth, either on the board, or the floor, using sheets of paper or a series of cards (with stages of labour written on them) lined up.

Group members select a card listing one of the interventions, drugs or obstetric procedures. They then place this card on the time line at the appropriate place. There may be more than one card with a complication, for example, there could be several cards saying 'fetal distress' or 'failure to progress'.

The group then uses lengths of string or coloured wool, or draws lines on the board, to link the various procedures:

- induction linked to epidural, forceps, episiotomy
- fetal distress linked to electronic fetal monitoring, caesarean or forceps and episiotomy
- failure to progress linked to artificial rupture of membranes, epidural, oxytocin drip, vacuum extraction

Encourage the group to make as many links as possible, and there are many variations that could eventuate. Have lots of string or wool available.

POINTS TO WATCH

☛ Try to encourage the group to find positive outcomes for interventions, not just negative ones. Sometimes a timely intervention will save lives.

☛ Have cards which also cover the early post-partum period as well ('Baby in special care nursery', 'Baby slow to suck in the first few days', 'Increased risk of jaundice' etc.).

FURTHER READING

Balaskas J. 1989, *The New Active Birth*, Harper Collins.

Baldwin R. & Palmarini T. 1986, *Pregnant feelings: developing trust in birth*, Celestial Arts, California, USA.

Fisher R. & Ury W. 1991, *Getting to Yes*, Random Century.

Geldard D. 1993, *Basic Personal Counselling*, Prentice Hall.

Hamer K. 1991, *Leading a Group*, Kerry Hamer, Sydney.

Hunter D., Bailey A. & Taylor B. 1992, *The Zen of Groups*, Tandem Press, New Zealand.

Ilse S. 1992, *Empty Arms*, Wintergreen Press, USA.

Kitzinger S. 1979, *Education and Counselling for Childbirth*, Balliere Tindall, London.

McKay S. 1986, *The Assertive Approach to Childbirth*, ICEA, Minneapolis, USA.

Nicol M. *Loss of a Baby: Understanding Maternal Grief*, Bantam.

Peckham D. 1988, *ICEA Guide for Childbirth Educators*, ICEA, Minneapolis, USA.

Robertson A. 1990, *Your Childbirth Education Classes: finding clients*, ACE Graphics, Sydney, Australia.

Robertson A. 1990, *Making Birth Easier*, ACE Graphics, Sydney, Australia.

Robertson A. 1994, *Preparing for Birth*, Ace Graphics, Sydney, Australia.

Rogers J. 1989, *Adults Learning*, Open University Press, United Kingdom.

SANDS UK 1991, *Miscarriage Stillbirth and Neonatal Death — a guide for health professionals*, SANDS UK.

Small H. 1991, *Icebreakers and Warm Ups*, Parents Centres New Zealand.

Szirom T. & Dyson S. 1985, *Greater Expectations*, YWCA of Australia, Melbourne.

The Clarity Collective 1983, *Taught not Caught*, Spiral Educational Resources, Australia.

Part 4

Putting it all together

Chapter 9

Designing your pre-natal classes

In this manual we have concentrated on the major theme of pre-natal classes, that is, teaching about normal physiology of labour, and ways of achieving an active birth. There are many other subjects that can be included, and you need to find a way of weaving the whole content together into a cohesive, positive story that empowers your clients to have confidence in themselves and their ability to birth naturally. In this chapter we will look at ways of devising a teaching plan for your entire class series, even though some of the topics may not have been covered extensively in this manual.

A simple planning strategy for classes involves focusing on *what* and *why* we are teaching (content), with *whom* we will be working (target group), *when* will the group gather (format), *where* will the group meet (venue) and *how* will we teach (presentation and teaching method).

What will we teach?

There is a vast amount of information that could be included in pre-natal classes. Childbirth educators usually have an extensive background knowledge about birth and parenting, are keen to enthuse others about birth, and are anxious that parents make decisions based on detailed information about the options available. Parents, on the other hand, may have some information already, are usually keen to know more, but equally may not want all the facts, since this may be scary, or just impossible to remember.

As an educator, you need to develop a means of sifting through the mountain of facts at your disposal to select the information needed by your clients at any given time. Overloading them may cause confusion, and giving detailed explanations of medical procedures, for example, may enhance fears or tip the perspective of the classes towards the abnormal. In addition, many parents are blissfully ignorant through lack of experience and so can offer few clues about what they need. Therefore, how do we decide what to teach?

Firstly, we need to discover what parents know already. There are many ways this can be done, both at the beginning of the class series, and regularly throughout, as new topics are introduced. There are some ideas on how to do this in Part 3 of this book.

Secondly, we know that parents will need information in certain areas, specifically related to pregnancy, the birth process and its management, the post-partum period and parenting. It is part of our job to introduce this information to prospective parents so they can be better prepared for what may lie ahead. We have a responsibility to alert parents to situations they are likely to encounter, even though our inability to predict outcomes will not allow us to prepare parents for every eventuality.

In combining these two aspects, we need some basic beliefs:

- Every woman has a right to know what is happening to her and her baby, and to be involved in making decisions that may affect them both.
- Mothers want to protect their babies and do everything possible to ensure a safe outcome during birth.
- It is possible for every woman to gain the information she needs: the challenge is for educators to communicate effectively so the message is understood. No parent should be labelled as 'too stupid' to understand. If the message has not been received, then the problem lies with us, the educators, not our clients.

In terms of what to teach, begin with what people already know, and add extra information when they indicate they want or need it. To avoid burdening them with unnecessary facts, start with the basic essentials and use their questions as clues to the extra detail they want. If you encourage a healthy curiosity about these topics (and this is not difficult, since parents are usually very keen to know as much as possible) you will quickly discover where to add extra detail.

In some areas, such as parenting, there are more potential areas for discussion than available time in the average pre-natal class group. Therefore, some negotiation will be necessary, to decide what to include and which information will need to be obtained elsewhere or at another time.

At all times, when considering what to teach, put the needs of your clients first. It may be difficult for group members to describe their specific needs at the beginning of the class series, but if you take a learner-centred, problem-solving approach to leading the group, rather than a traditional 'teacher' role, your clients will soon feel comfortable asking for information. Encouraging parents to find their own solutions for problems is a basic premise of these classes, and part of this process involves them seeking the facts they need prior to making decisions. Of course, their needs will change as the pregnancy advances, or if the circumstances surrounding their health care changes and as they learn more in the group. This is one reason why beginning classes with a tightly structured program can create problems: the group's needs may change, and you therefore need flexibility in your class outline, to renegotiate the agenda, check for progress and consult with the group before changing your approach as necessary.

When considering what the group *wants*, however, you also need to include information and skill building exercises you know the group *needs*. Not only to do you have to consider how to supply the resources and information the group have requested, but you also have a responsibility to ensure they have details and facts that they need in order to fully consider an issue. For example, you may be asked about pain relieving drugs for labour. Group members may know little about the specific drugs involved, so you have a responsibility to tell them about all the alternatives. Even if they don't ask about possible side effects, you must include these details so that they receive a complete picture of the options available. Similarly, knowing the facts is not very useful unless your client has practised communication skills, including negotiation and compromising.

In summary, learning what to include and leave out in a class series takes time and experience. Initially, plan to include the basic topics you know to be of interest to expectant parents, and information you are aware they will need when making decisions about their care. Plan to keep this information brief and present it in an interesting way that will excite, inform and arouse curiosity. Leave yourself time to explore other issues nominated by the group and to answer questions generated by your presentation. A flexible program, where you can change your topics around as needed will give you confidence, and help you avoid feelings of stress if the classes become rearranged. All the time, include your group in the planning of their classes, and keep their needs ahead of your own.

WHY ARE WE TEACHING THESE TOPICS?

Having decided the basic outline, the next step is to consider why we are including them. For what reason have we listed them in the program? What is our purpose in allocating time for this particular issue? In addition, what do we expect our clients will get from considering this topic? What do we want them to achieve by discussing these issues?

As you answer these questions, you will be devising a set of aims and objectives for your teaching. Ways to prepare objectives have been covered in an earlier chapter in this book. Now that you are actively planning your classes, you need to prepare learning objectives for all the topics in the class series and teaching objectives that identify how you will set about achieving the learning objectives you have listed.

This process will take time, but when complete you will have a very clear idea of what you will be doing in the classes, and a sense of purpose, clearly described, that will allow you to introduce the flexible approach necessary for effective learning. This may seem a paradox: a very structured program that allows flexibility! In practice, when you know exactly what you are trying to achieve and have a written plan of both the learning objectives for your clients and teaching strategies for yourself, introducing flexibility into the class format becomes easier. You know that you can cover a particular topic either in this session, or next week. You know that your learning objective can be reached by trying either activity (a), perhaps geared for more visual learners, or through activity (b), designed to appeal to auditory learners. Sometimes you may discover that you can reach your learning objective by travelling down a completely different path, or that an activity designed for one learning objective can be easily adapted to meet another. Having a clear sense of what you are trying to achieve makes these interesting and exciting discoveries more likely, and it is these unexpected insights that add challenge and thrill to working with adults.

Who will be our clients?

There are several aspects to this question. Firstly, you need to consider your target audience. Will you be working with a group who have similar, perhaps special, needs? Pre-natal groups for teenagers, single mothers, ethnic community groups, high risk women in an antenatal hospital ward, highly educated middle class achievers, second time mothers or women who have had previous caesarean sections, are all examples of groups with a special focus.

Secondly, each individual within the group will also have special needs, regardless of their primary reason for joining the group. We need to consider both of these aspects when planning and presenting our classes.

Perhaps you have advertised your classes to reach a particular group of pregnant women, and therefore the group is reasonably homogeneous. Sometimes this will happen easily — for example, working with a group of 'high-risk' women admitted to hospital to await the birth of their babies. Although these women have much in common, especially the label 'high-risk', they are still individuals, in that their medical conditions may vary, and their personal backgrounds will be different. Working from a basis of the common needs of these women, a particular program can be devised, with allowances for specific needs. This kind of focused group makes planning relatively easy.

Many pre-natal groups, however, will not have strong common bonds based on similar backgrounds or circumstances. Most groups are a mixture of individuals, often with very different goals, attitudes, backgrounds and beliefs. Planning for these groups will require a broader perspective, with group negotiation to identify those issues that are of interest to everyone. It will be difficult to meet the needs of every individual within your group, unless it is kept small (a maximum of 20 people), and sufficient time can be allocated to each meeting (a minimum of 2 hours for each session, plus breaks).

WHEN WILL WE PRESENT THE CLASSES?

This question raises several points for consideration: the timing of the classes in the pregnancy, the format to be used and the specific hour of day to be set aside for the group's meetings.

Learning is more efficient if the material being addressed is relevant to the learner at the time or if it can be used immediately as reinforcement for the learning. Traditionally, pre-natal classes have consisted of a series of six or eight weekly sessions usually timed for the last trimester of pregnancy. Yet pregnant women need information and support earlier than this, and much information about baby care will be forgotten before it can be used. Perhaps it is time to reconsider this approach to scheduling pre-natal groups and instead to devise a program that is timed differently. Try asking yourself:

- Is the information I want to include relevant to the learners at this time in their pregnancy?
- Will the information be useful now?
- What would be an appropriate time to cover the topics on my list?

There are many possible formats for pre-natal classes. Experimenting will provide diversity and challenge in your teaching, and selecting an appropriate format may make it easier to attract your target audience. You could consider:

TYPES OF CLASSES

- Break the eight week format into three:
  — Two early pregnancy classes (12–16 weeks)
  — Two parenting classes (around 26–28 weeks)
  — Four birth classes (34–38 weeks)
- Post-natal parenting classes

- Class reunions
- Classes for first time parents
- Refresher groups for parents with other children
- Mixed classes for first-time and experienced parents
- Single sex classes, or a special night for the men and women separately
- Classes for women with special needs or a special focus (single parents, 'high risk' women, pregnant teenagers, women with similar cultural backgrounds, Vaginal Birth After Caesarean classes etc.)

AVAILABILITY OF CLASSES

- Daytime classes
- Night time classes
- Week days/nights
- Weekends
- Weekly classes
- Workshops over several consecutive days

COMPOSITION OF THE GROUP

- Casual 'drop-in' classes
- Scheduled groups
- Same group members for the whole series
- 'Revolving door' classes for whoever arrives for the session
- Small groups
- Large groups
- Individual counselling/private consultations

You can see there are many potential combinations! Varying your groups will keep you fresh and avoid educator burnout. The stimulation of trying something different will assist your professional development and add further dimensions to your work.

Choosing a suitable time for the classes is also important. People in full time employment may like to attend a group straight after work to avoid a trip home, a hurried meal then going out again. Alternatively, others may need to eat before they come, to help them stay awake! Weekend groups, either as a compact workshop or spread over a number of consecutive weekends may have appeal for working parents or those with other children, who find leaving the children with relatives easier for one weekend rather than for shorter times spread over a longer period. Daytime sessions might be useful for shift workers, and may be essential for ethnic communities where women do not venture out at night.

In all cases it may be possible to arrange the first session and then negotiate the meeting times for the remainder of the series with the group itself. Many pregnant women are tired at night, especially if they are working outside the home and/or have other children.

WHERE WILL WE TEACH?

Choosing a suitable venue is important. Some pointers for selecting venues are included in chapter 3. The location may be especially relevant if you are targeting a particular group. Pre-natal classes have often been held in health facilities, such as a hospital or community health centre. This could tend to emphasise the medical model in the minds of some potential participants or may be an inappropriate gathering place for many others. You may achieve better attendance if you locate the classes in a neutral setting or one that is closely linked with the group you wish to attract. Taking the classes out to the people is also a better strategy than expecting them to always come to you.

Some educators use their own homes as a venue. This certainly creates the right kind of social atmosphere for the group, and can work well providing that you have space and it is not disruptive to your family.

Other educators have chosen venues for their particular attributes: a meeting room in a resort hotel for a weekend group aimed at working parents, a room in the community centre for the young unemployed as a means of reaching teenagers, a church hall for women of a particular ethnic group.

Whatever venue you choose you will need to be sure that it has the facilities you need, is comfortable, and has a suitable space for the activities you are planning. It may be necessary for you to sign a contract for its use, and you will need insurance to cover breakage of equipment and accidents on the premises. Public liability insurance will usually cover these eventualities. Professional indemnity insurance is not considered necessary for childbirth educators, since educators are not treating clients, diagnosing problems, giving advice or prescribing. Your role is to offer information and teach skills which are used by your clients to make their own decisions and to take responsibility for their own actions. You do have a professional responsibility to ensure that the information is accurate, not biased or misleading. Any exercises you teach must be correctly demonstrated, and you should check that they have been understood, especially if clients are to practise unsupervised at home.

How will we teach?

As we have discovered, presenting a pre-natal class is more than standing in front of a group and talking. Deciding how to teach involves decisions about the presentation method you will use, choosing appropriate teaching strategies, planning a suitable format, selecting useful teaching aids and evaluating the outcome.

Presentation ideas and specific teaching strategies have already been described elsewhere in this book. Setting out your teaching plan is a vital step in preparing for your group, and is worthy of time and careful consideration. The following suggestions are based on a series of eight classes, spread over the pregnancy, beginning with two early pregnancy groups, followed by two parenting groups and four classes focusing on the birth and immediate post-partum period. You will need to adapt these ideas for your own group, and this outline is intended only as a guide, to illustrate the planning process.

Preparation for birth and parenting classes

For the series as a whole

- Global aims
- Learner objectives

Throughout the whole series

- Emphasis on consistent, congruent themes
- Reinforcement of main messages through multiple practice sessions
- Inter-weaving the information to highlight the continuum of pregnancy, birth and parenting
- Attention to specific needs of clients
- Skills development encouraged through participation in appropriate activities
- Counselling not teaching

Topics to be covered

- Early pregnancy classes
  - nutrition
  - taking care of yourself: exercise, discomforts etc.
  - emotional/physical changes
  - choosing caregivers and the place of birth
  - medical tests and pregnancy care
  - premature labour and pregnancy complications

- Parenting classes
  - adjusting lifestyles
  - changing relationships: roles, sexual, shared parenting etc.
  - about newborns: characteristics, developmental milestones
  - baby care equipment: layette, safety etc.
  - breastfeeding
  - complications: sick babies etc.
- Birth and early post-partum
  - stages of labour: anatomy and physiology
  - self-help measures
  - role of support people
  - complications
  - drugs and medical interventions
  - beginning breastfeeding
  - maternal post-partum recovery
  - unforeseen outcomes

FOR EACH OF THESE BROAD TOPICS

- learning objectives for clients
- teaching objectives
  - focused on skills development
  - in at least 3 different modes (visual, auditory, kinaesthetic)
  - including strategies for different learning styles (linear/lateral; big picture/jigsaw; passive/experiential)
- content points listed
- teaching equipment listed
- evaluation method described

FOR EACH CLASS OR SESSION

- broad topics identified
- teaching activities varied e.g. whole group discussion followed by exercise session, then small groups followed by a video and discussion etc.
- a variety of teaching aids used
- change of activity every 20–30 minutes
- suitable break for refreshments around the middle of the session
- time allocated for introductions at the beginning and summarising at the end

After each session

- post-class evaluation
- listing of topics included/ left out
- rearranging of next class to include missed topics or to include requested information

At the end of the series

- full evaluation of educator and client outcomes
- incorporation of feedback into planning for the next series
- post-natal reunion, to conclude the group process

Choosing teaching aids

It is important that your philosophy on birth be consistent throughout the class series if you are to avoid confusing your message. Choosing appropriate audiovisual aids that reinforce a positive attitude and enhance confidence requires care. There can be no doubt that using good teaching equipment can enliven any presentation and enhance learning, and having a variety of materials will allow you to choose an appropriate medium that suits your group. The list of possible teaching aids is extensive:

- charts
- white or blackboard
- felt board
- paper and pens, pencils
- overhead transparencies
- slides
- drawings, cartoons
- photographs
- samples of equipment (cord clamps, hot packs, EFM printouts etc.)
- music
- videos
- audiotapes (crying baby, labour sounds etc.)
- models (pelvis, fetal doll, knitted uterus etc.)
- your own body (positions for labour etc.)
- labour ward tour
- real babies!
- real mothers!

In addition to these pieces of 'hardware', remember that teaching strategies such as demonstrations, story telling, role playing, game playing, quizzes, analogies etc. all form part of the 'software' for teaching, and can also be included under the heading of teaching aids.

When making your selection, there are several points worth considering:

- Look for variety. Every topic could be covered using of a number of different teaching aids.

- Choose quality products that will resist damage and look good for many years. Teaching equipment can be expensive, so investing in hard-wearing and multi-purpose aids makes sense.

- Charts, drawings or diagrams with no writing on them are more useful than illustrations with captions, that must be explained. All you need is the picture — you can then add whatever words or description is appropriate.

- Some home-made teaching aids can be fun and inventive, but too many will detract from your professional image.

- Charts or other illustrations for class use must be large enough for the group to see easily. Small writing, pastel colours and too much detail can be frustrating and distracting.

- Printed material should be easy to read, well presented and written in suitable language. Check printed handouts for jargon, unnecessary medical terminology and messages reinforcing the medical model of childbirth.

- Illustrations should reflect your message. If you have been discussing the benefits of upright birth, avoid using pictures that show women giving birth lying down. This will undermine your credibility, cause confusion and reinforce the medical view of birth.

- Models should be easy to use and sturdy. Practise using them in advance, in front of a mirror to check how they will appear to your audience.

- Handle your fetal doll and pelvis with care and reverence. Your clients may be distressed if you casually throw your doll around or handle the pelvis carelessly.

- Some teaching aids have more predictable learning outcomes than others. For example, it is hard to misunderstand a well-illustrated chart. Videos, on the other hand, are open to many interpretations, as are demonstrations, audiotapes, stories and analogies. This does not mean that you should avoid using these teaching media because you cannot predict how they will be received, it just means that you must be prepared for a variety of reactions and responses whenever you present them.

- Always view videos in advance so you know their content. There is no need to necessarily show the whole tape — smaller clips could be used to allow time to show a greater variety of labours.
- Not everyone wants, or needs, to see a birth video. Obtain the group's permission before you screen them and schedule the video session so that those who want to leave can do so without feeling embarrassed or missing post-video information.

It is not essential to have a vast array of teaching aids to run effective pre-natal classes. With a little skill and lateral thinking, an educator can use her own body for many demonstrations, and encourage couples to use their own bodies to get in touch with the baby and to work out what is happening during pregnancy and labour. Too many charts and too many gadgets can be a distraction and lead to a reliance on props which distances you from your class. Choose a few basic teaching aids initially, and only add to your collection when you feel a particular teaching aid would definitely benefit your presentation. Remember that experiential learning and involvement of the group in active participation is often the most effective way for adults to learn.

EVALUATION

Evaluation is an essential part of any teaching process. When you plan your class series you should also plan the way in which you will receive feedback from your clients about the effectiveness of your work. Evaluation can be done in a number of different ways: continuously through each class ('Is my message getting through?'); at the end of each class ('Have I achieved my objectives for this session?'); at the end of the series, before the birth ('Did we fulfil the overall aims for the series?' 'Did my clients achieve their objectives in coming to class?'); and after the birth. Details of evaluation procedures have been described earlier with suggestions for specific activities outlined in Part 3. Some further suggestions for more global evaluation methods are described below.

QUESTIONNAIRES

Many educators use surveys or questionnaires completed by their clients after the birth of their baby as a basic form of evaluation. Questions on these surveys should not only focus on yes/no answers but should also allow for specific feedback about their experiences and the value of the classes as a preparation tool. People often have difficulty telling an educator directly, or even indirectly, if there were aspects of the classes that they found unsatisfactory. Include the potential for negative feedback as part of the questionnaire itself, as this is a most useful form of evaluation for reviewing your content and teaching style. Anonymous questionnaires may make it easier for clients to offer honest comment.

Many educators like to collect these evaluations at the last pre-natal class, but a better time may be at the reunion, when the true value of their pre-natal education can be more objectively assessed.

Referrals

Sources of referral form another useful evaluation tool. Satisfied customers are your best advertisement, so recommendations made by former clients are an indication that they valued your efforts. Referrals from doctors and hospitals can also give useful feedback, although be aware that sometimes doctors, in particular, recommend classes because they regard them as non-controversial and 'safe'. If your classes are viewed this way by other health professionals then you may wish to review your presentation and content to ensure that it does not reinforce the medical model for birth.

Attending births

Going to births yourself as a support person is one of the most effective ways of assessing whether what you are teaching has relevance and practical benefit for your clients. Attending births can also form part of your own ongoing education, and all educators should try to attend as many births as possible. If you attend births with an open mind and a willingness to learn from the labouring woman, then you will gain not only much useful insight into the labouring process, but you will discover many practical tips and suggestions you can add to your class content. It will also help to broaden your outlook and to widen your understanding of the many ways in which women labour and give birth.

Over to you . . .

Having worked through the theory outlined in this book, now is the time to put it to practical use. Just as there are no formulas for giving birth, there are no formulas for perfect pre-natal classes. Parents leave your group to make their own way through the birth process, so now you must learn from experience and discover for yourselves the pleasures and rewards of working with expectant parents. Pre-natal education can be a powerful tool in the empowerment of women, and may be pivotal in helping them, and their partners, achieve the birth experience of their choice.

Teaching resources

Associates in Childbirth Education

10 Mallett Street (PO Box 366)
Camperdown NSW 2050
Australia
Phone: +61 2 516 3077
Fax: +61 2 516 1040

For training courses in childbirth education including the Graduate Diploma in Childbirth Education.

ACE Graphics (Australia)

10 Mallett Street (PO Box 366)
Camperdown NSW 2050
Australia
Phone: +61 2 516 3077
Fax: +61 2 516 1040

For teaching aids — charts, models, videotapes, audiotapes and professional reference books and leaflets. Mail order service to anywhere in the world.

ACE Graphics (United Kingdom)

PO Box 173
Sevenoaks Kent
United Kingdom
TN14 7EZ
Phone: +44 959 524 622
Fax: +44 959 524 622

For teaching aids — charts, models, videotapes, audiotapes and professional reference books and leaflets. Mail order service to anywhere in the world.

Childbirth Graphics (A division of WRS Group)

PO Box 21207
Waco TX 76702-9964
USA
Phone: +1 800 299 3366 (within the USA)
Fax: +1 817 751 0221

For teaching aids — charts, models, videotapes, audiotapes within the USA and Canada.

INTERNATIONAL CHILDBIRTH EDUCATION ASSOCIATION

ICEA Bookcenter
PO Box 20048
Minneapolis Minnesota 55420
USA
Phone:+1 800 624 4934 (within the USA)
Fax: +1 612 854 8772

For books and reference materials related to childbirth education.

THE ACTIVE BIRTH CENTRE

55 Dartmouth Park Road
London NW5 1SL
Phone: +44 71 267 3006
Fax: +44 71 267 5368

For information about active birth, video and audiotapes.

THE COCHRANE COLLABORATION PREGNANCY & CHILDBIRTH DATABASE

Update Software Ltd
Manor Cottage, Little Milton
Oxford OX44 7QB
United Kingdom
Phone: +44 844 278 887
Fax: +44 844 278 887

ACE Graphics (Australian agent)
PO Box 366
Camperdown NSW 2050
Australia
Phone: +61 2 516 3077
Fax: +61 2 516 1040

A computer database extending the information contained in *Effective care in Pregnancy in Childbirth*, containing 600 regularly updated systematic reviews of the effects of care in pregnancy and childbirth compiled by the Cochrane Collaboration in Oxford.

Midwives Information and Resource Service (MIDIRS)

9 Elmdale Rd
Clifton
Bristol BS8 1SL
United Kingdom
Phone: +44 272 251 791
Fax: +44 272 251 792

ACE Graphics (Australian agent)
PO Box 366
Camperdown NSW 2050
Australia
Phone: +61 2 516 3077
Fax: +61 2 516 1040

Subscription service, published four times a year, of news, views and research from the world of midwifery, gathered from over 450 international sources.

Index